PE Workbook
100 Workouts
2021

N. Rey | darebee.com

First Printing, 2021

ISBN 13: 978-1-84481-165-6
ISBN 10: 1-84481-165-4

Warning and Disclaimer
Although every precaution has been taken to verify the accuracy of the information contained herein, the author and publisher assume no responsibility for any errors or omissions. No liability is assumed for damage or injury that may result from the use of information contained within.

Workouts

1. Action Hero
2. Aladdin
3. Andromeda
4. Arms & Back
5. Aurora
6. Baby Steps
7. Bard
8. Below Zero
9. Best Shot
10. Best Thing
11. Big Bang
12. Breathless
13. Cant Stop Me Now
14. Cardio & Coordination
15. Cardio Circuit
16. Cardio Fusion
17. Cardio Shock
18. Chapter One
19. Chisel
20. Climber
21. Cronus
22. Crusher
23. Dragon Reborn
24. Easy Does It
25. Everyday Hero
26. Explorer
27. Extractor
28. Extra Mile
29. Falcon
30. Floor Is Lava
31. Frost
32. Fundamentals
33. Gambit
34. Goblin
35. Golem
36. Grade A
37. Gravity
38. Guardian
39. Hall Of Fame
40. Here & Now
41. Hermit
42. Hero
43. High Burn
44. Hit The Ground
45. Ice Age
46. Journeyman
47. Journey
48. Kinder
49. Knight
50. Launchpad
51. Lazy Bear
52. Level Up
53. Lifeguard
54. Low Impact
55. Mage
56. Make My Day
57. Maverick
58. Mediator
59. Move It, Move It
60. Never Give Up
61. Next Level
62. No Capes
63. No Sweat Cardio
64. Overlap
65. Perfect 10
66. Power Cardio
67. Power Circuit
68. Power Run
69. Protagonist
70. Protector
71. Push-Up Party
72. Raw Grit
73. Regenerator
74. Roaster
75. Rocking Around
76. Rookie
77. Roundabout
78. Sage
79. Shapeshifter
80. So Far So Good
81. Spaceman
82. Spartan
83. Stand & Tall
84. Step One
85. Stopgap
86. Story Mode
87. Super Easy
88. Superstar
89. Temple Run
90. Top Of The World
91. Total Blast
92. Track & Field
93. Tracker
94. Triathlete
95. Up & Down
96. Upgrade
97. Upperbody
98. Victory Lap
99. Watchman
100. White Rabbit

The Manual

Workout posters are read from left to right and contain the following information: grid with exercises (images), number of reps (repetitions) next to each, number of sets for your fitness level (I, II or III) and rest time.

SAMPLE WORKOUT

LEVEL I 3 sets LEVEL II 5 sets LEVEL III 7 sets REST up to 2 minutes

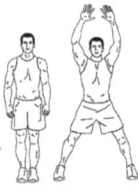

10 jumping jacks

20 high knes

40 side-to-side chops

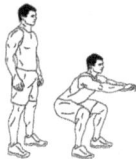 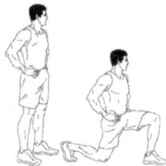

10 squats

20 lunges

10-count plank

20 climbers

10 plank jump-ins

to failure push-ups

Difficulty Levels:

Level I: normal

Level II: hard

Level III: advanced

1 set

10 jumping jacks

20 high knees (10 each leg)

40 side-to-side chops (20 each side)

10 squats

20 lunges (10 each leg)

10-count plank (hold while counting to 10)

20 climbers (10 each leg)

10 plank jump-ins

to failure push-ups (your maximum)

Up to 2 minutes rest between sets

30 seconds, 60 seconds or 2 minutes - it's up to you.

"Reps" stands for repetitions, how many times an exercise is performed. Reps are usually located next to each exercise's name. Number of reps is always a total number for both legs / arms / sides. It's easier to count this way: e.g. if it says 20 climbers, it means that both legs are already counted in - it is 10 reps each leg.

Reps to failure means to muscle failure = your personal maximum, you repeat the move until you can't. It can be anything from one rep to twenty, normally applies to more challenging exercises. The goal is to do as many as you possibly can.

The transition from exercise to exercise is an important part of each circuit (set) - it is often what makes a particular workout more effective. Transitions are carefully worked out to hyperload specific muscle groups more for better results. For example if you see a plank followed by push-ups it means that you start performing push-ups right after you finished with the plank avoiding dropping your body on the floor in between.

There is no rest between exercises - only after sets, unless specified otherwise. You have to complete the entire set going from one exercise to the next as fast as you can before you can rest.

What does "up to 2 minutes rest" mean: it means you can rest for up to 2 minutes but the sooner you can go again the better. Eventually your recovery time will improve naturally, you won't need all two minutes to recover - and that will also be an indication of your improving fitness.

Recommended rest time:

Level I: 2 minutes or less
Level II: 60 seconds or less
Level III: 30 seconds or less

Video Exercise Library
http://darebee.com/video

The workouts are organized in alphabetical order so you can find the workouts you favor easier and faster.

Introduction

Bodyweight training may look easy, but if you are not used to it, it's very far from that. It is just as intense as running and it is just as challenging so if you struggle with it at the very beginning, it's perfectly ok – you will get better at it once you start doing it regularly. Do it at your own pace and take longer breaks if you need to.

You can start with a single individual workout from the collection and see how you feel. If you are new to bodyweight training always start any workout on Level I (level of difficulty).

You can pick any number of workouts per week, usually between 3 and 5 and rotate them for maximum results.

warmup

by DAREBEE © darebee.com
Repeat each exercise for 10-20 seconds then move on to the next one.

#1

NOTES

date

_____

total time

_____

set counter

☐ ☐ ☐ ☐ ☐ ☐ ☐

ACTION HERO

DAREBEE WORKOUT
© darebee.com

LEVEL I 3 sets
LEVEL II 5 sets
LEVEL III 7 sets
REST up to 2 minutes

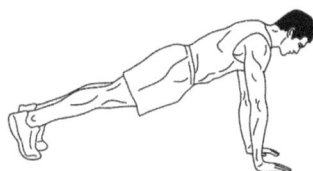

10-count plank

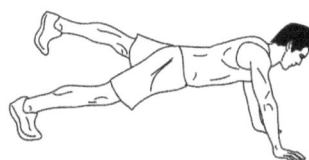

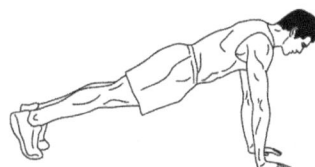

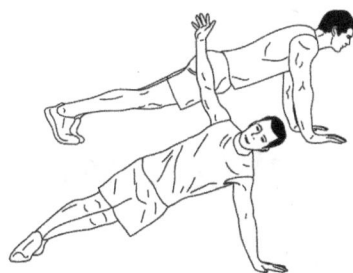

10 plank leg raises

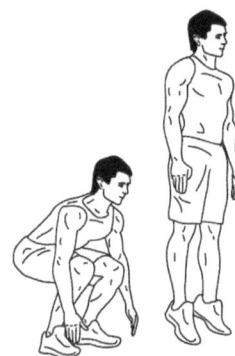

4 jump squats

10-count plank

4 push-ups

10 bicep extensions

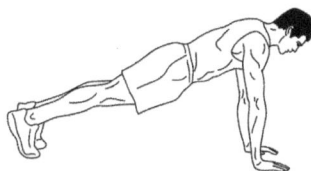

10-count plank

10 plank rotations

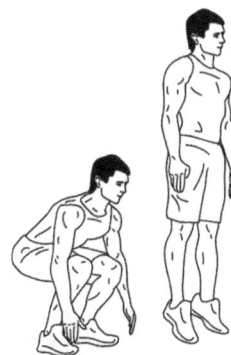

4 jump squats

#2

NOTES

date

_____

total time

_____

set counter

☐ ☐ ☐ ☐ ☐ ☐ ☐

ALADDIN

DAREBEE WORKOUT © darebee.com

LEVEL I 3 sets **LEVEL II** 5 sets **LEVEL III** 7 sets **REST** up to 2 minutes

10 jumping jacks

4 jumping lunges

10 jumping jacks

10 shoulder taps

4 burpees

10 shoulder taps

10 jumping jacks

4 jumping lunges

10 jumping jacks

#3

NOTES

date

_____

total time

_____

set counter

☐ ☐ ☐ ☐ ☐ ☐ ☐

Andromeda

DAREBEE WORKOUT © darebee.com

LEVEL I 3 sets **LEVEL II** 5 sets **LEVEL III** 7 sets **REST** up to 2 minutes

10 wide squats

10 squat hold side bends

10 plank leg raises

10 plank rotations

10-count plank hold

10 bridges

4 single leg bridges

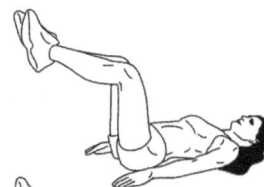

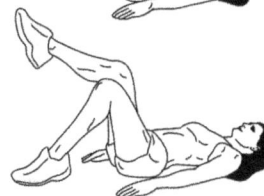

10 toe taps

#4
NOTES

date

_____

total time

_____

set counter

☐ ☐ ☐ ☐ ☐ ☐ ☐

arms
&back

WORKOUT BY
© darebee.com

LEVEL I 3 sets
LEVEL II 5 sets
LEVEL III 7 sets
REST up to 2 minutes

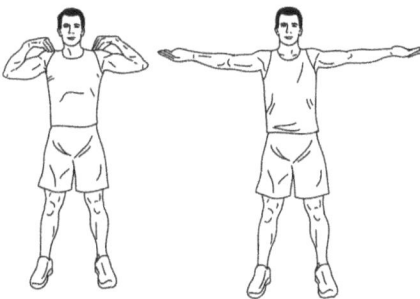

20 side bicep extensions

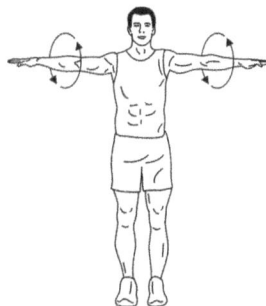

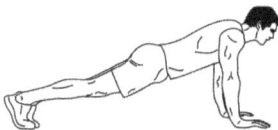

20 raised arm circles

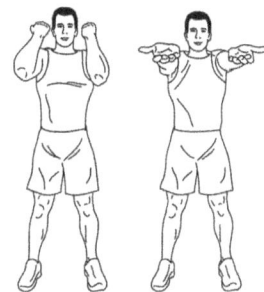

20 bicep extensions

10 shoulder taps

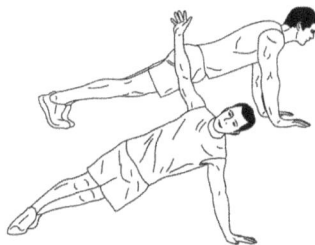

10 plank rotations

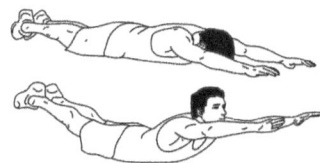

10 superman stretches

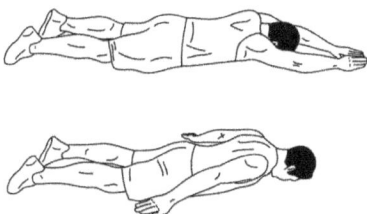

10 reverse angels

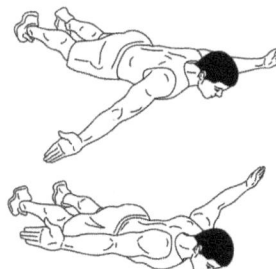

10 prone reverse flys

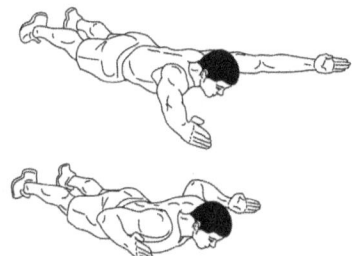

10 W-extensions

#5

NOTES

date

_____

total time

_____

set counter

☐ ☐ ☐ ☐ ☐ ☐ ☐

AURORA

DAREBEE WORKOUT © darebee.com

LEVEL I 3 sets **LEVEL II** 5 sets **LEVEL III** 7 sets **REST** up to 2 minutes

20 march steps

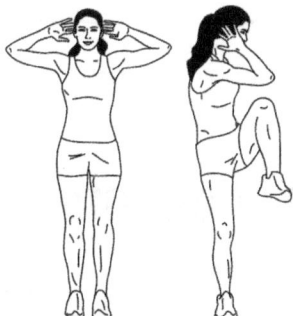

10 knee-to-elbows

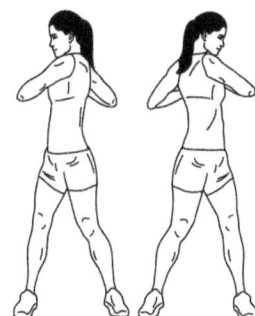

10 side leg raises

20 march steps

10 knee-to-elbows

10 calf raises

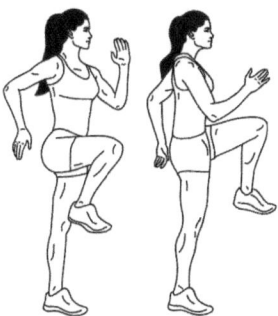

20 march steps

10 knee-to-elbows

10 torso rotations

#6

NOTES

date

_____

total time

_____

set counter

□ □ □ □ □ □ □

BABY STEPS

DAREBEE WORKOUT
© darebee.com
LEVEL I 3 sets
LEVEL II 5 sets
LEVEL III 7 sets
REST up to 2 minutes

10 march steps

10 scissor chops

10 arm scissors

10 march steps

10 chest expansions

10 arm circles

#7

NOTES

date

_____

total time

_____

set counter

☐ ☐ ☐ ☐ ☐ ☐ ☐

THE BARD

DAREBEE WORKOUT © darebee.com

LEVEL I 3 sets **LEVEL II** 5 sets **LEVEL III** 7 sets **REST** up to 2 minutes

20 butt kicks   **20** high knees   **10** climbers

20 butt kicks   **20** high knees   **10** shoulder taps

#8
NOTES

date

_____

total time

_____

set counter

☐ ☐ ☐ ☐ ☐ ☐ ☐

Below Zero

DAREBEE WORKOUT © darebee.com

LEVEL I 3 sets **LEVEL II** 5 sets **LEVEL III** 7 sets **REST** up to 2 minutes

4 sit to stand

Hold on for support if needed

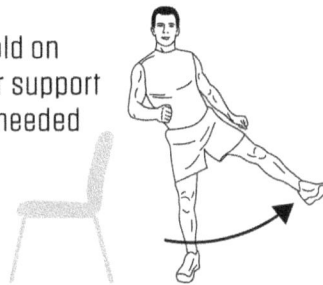

10 side leg raises

Hold on for support if needed

10 back leg raises

10 step jacks

4 side bends

4 hip rotations

10 bicep extensions

10 chest expansions

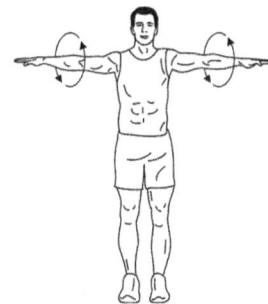

10 arm circles

#9

NOTES

date

_____

total time

_____

set counter

☐ ☐ ☐ ☐ ☐ ☐ ☐

MY BEST SHOT

DAREBEE WORKOUT © darebee.com

LEVEL I 3 sets **LEVEL II** 5 sets **LEVEL III** 7 sets **REST** up to 2 minutes

10 squat hops

10 bicep extensions

10 squat hops

10 butt kicks

10 squat hops

10 butt kicks

#10
NOTES

date

——————————

total time

——————————

set counter

☐ ☐ ☐ ☐ ☐ ☐ ☐

BEST THING
SINCE SLICED BREAD

DAREBEE
WORKOUT
© darebee.com
Level I 3 sets
Level II 5 sets
Level III 7 sets
2 minutes rest

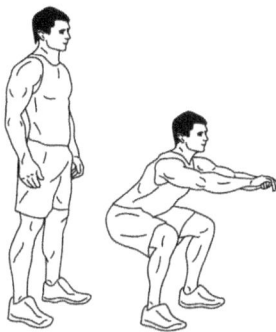

5 squats

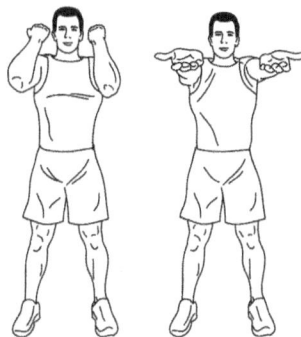

20 bicep extensions

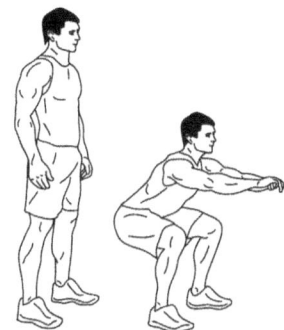

5 squats

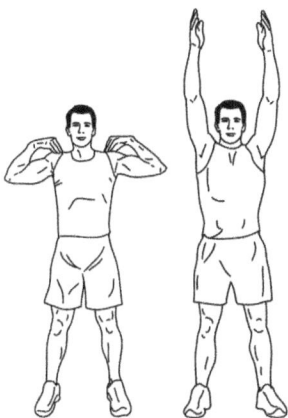

20 shoulder taps

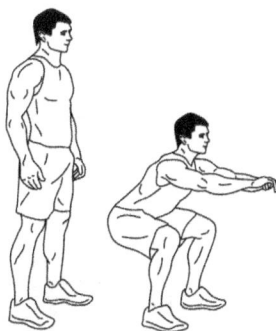

5 squats

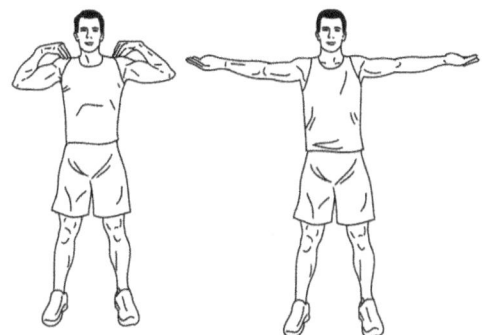

20 side shoulder taps

#11

NOTES

date

_____

total time

_____

set counter

☐ ☐ ☐ ☐ ☐ ☐ ☐

BIG BANG

DAREBEE WORKOUT
© darebee.com
LEVEL I 3 sets
LEVEL II 5 sets
LEVEL III 7 sets
REST up to 2 minutes

10 jumping jacks

2 push-ups

2 jump squats

10 jumping jacks

2 push-ups

2 plank jacks

10 jumping jacks

2 push-ups

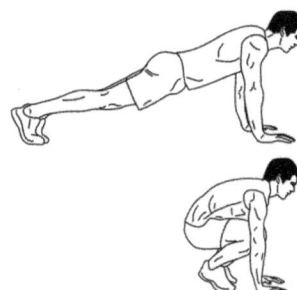

2 plank jump-ins

#12
NOTES

date

_____

total time

_____

set counter

☐ ☐ ☐ ☐ ☐ ☐ ☐

breathless

DAREBEE WORKOUT © darebee.com

LEVEL I 3 sets **LEVEL II** 5 sets **LEVEL III** 7 sets **REST** up to 2 minutes

20 high knees

2 jump squats

20 high knees

2 jumping lunges

20 high knees

2 jumping jacks

20 high knees

2 squat hops

20 high knees

#13
NOTES

date

_____

total time

_____

set counter

☐ ☐ ☐ ☐ ☐ ☐ ☐

CAN'T STOP ME NOW!

DAREBEE WORKOUT
© darebee.com
Level I 3 sets
Level II 5 sets
Level III 7 sets
2 minutes rest

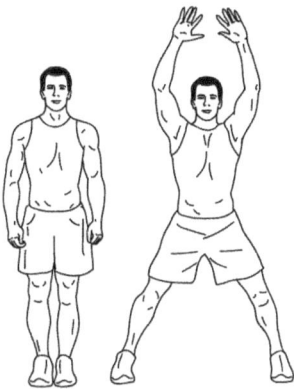

10 jumping jacks

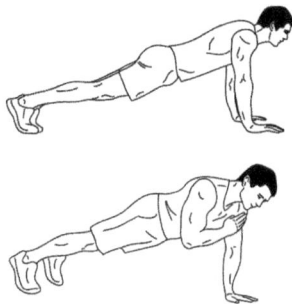

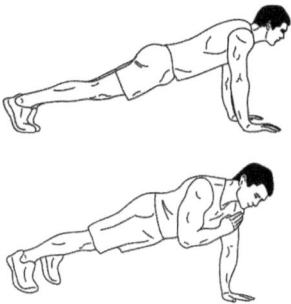

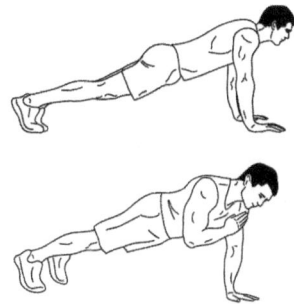

4 shoulder taps

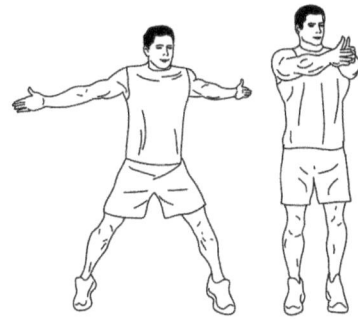

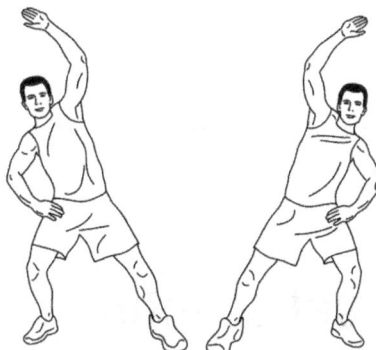

10 seal jacks

4 shoulder taps

10 side jacks

4 shoulder taps

#14
NOTES

date

_____

total time

_____

set counter

□ □ □ □ □ □ □

CARDIO &
COORDINATION

DAREBEE WORKOUT © darebee.com

LEVEL I 3 sets **LEVEL II** 5 sets **LEVEL III** 7 sets **REST** up to 2 minutes

10 butt kicks

6 single leg hops

10 butt kicks

10 jumping jacks

6 side-to-side jumps

10 jumping jacks

10 side leg raises

6 knee-to-elbows

10 side leg raises

#15

NOTES

date

_____

total time

_____

set counter

☐ ☐ ☐ ☐ ☐ ☐ ☐

CARDIO CIRCUIT

DAREBEE WORKOUT
© darebee.com
Level I 3 sets
Level II 5 sets
Level III 7 sets
2 minutes rest

10 seal jacks

4 jumping jacks

10 seal jacks

10 scissor chops

10 arm scissors

10 scissor chops

10 butt kicks

4 high knees

10 butt kicks

#16
NOTES

date

_____

total time

_____

set counter

□ □ □ □ □ □ □

CARDIO
FUSION

DAREBEE WORKOUT © darebee.com

LEVEL I 3 sets **LEVEL II** 5 sets **LEVEL III** 7 sets
REST up to 2 minutes

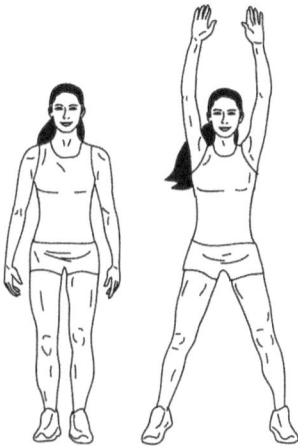

15 jumping jacks

10 side-to-side lunges

15 jumping jacks

10 raised arm circles

15 jumping jacks

10 twists

#17

NOTES

date

_____

total time

_____

set counter

☐ ☐ ☐ ☐ ☐ ☐ ☐

CARDIO
SHOCK

DAREBEE WORKOUT © darebee.com

LEVEL I 3 sets **LEVEL II** 5 sets **LEVEL III** 7 sets **REST** up to 2 minutes

20 jumping jacks

2 jump knee-tucks

20 jumping Ts

2 jump knee-tucks

20 seal jacks

2 jump knee-tucks

#18

NOTES

date

_____

total time

_____

set counter

☐ ☐ ☐ ☐ ☐ ☐ ☐

Chapter 1

DAREBEE WORKOUT © darebee.com

LEVEL I 3 sets **LEVEL II** 5 sets **LEVEL III** 7 sets **REST** up to 2 minutes

10 jumping jacks

6 squats

10 jumping jacks

10 march steps

10 jumping jacks

10 knee-to-elbow

10 jumping jacks

6 lunge step-up

10 jumping jacks

#19
NOTES

date

_____

total time

_____

set counter

☐ ☐ ☐ ☐ ☐ ☐ ☐

CHISEL

DAREBEE WORKOUT © darebee.com

LEVEL I 3 sets **LEVEL II** 5 sets **LEVEL III** 7 sets **REST** up to 2 minutes

20 high knees   **10** squats   **2** jump squats

20 high knees   **10** shoulder taps   **2** push-ups

20 high knees   **10** flutter kicks   **2** leg raises

#20
NOTES

date

_____

total time

_____

set counter

☐ ☐ ☐ ☐ ☐ ☐ ☐

THE CLIMBER

DAREBEE WORKOUT © darebee.com

LEVEL I 3 sets **LEVEL II** 5 sets **LEVEL III** 7 sets **REST** up to 2 minutes

20 climbers

4 push-ups

20 climbers

4 plank walk-outs

20 climbers

4 plank rotations

#21
NOTES

date

_____

total time

_____

set counter

☐ ☐ ☐ ☐ ☐ ☐ ☐

CRONUS

DAREBEE WORKOUT © darebee.com

LEVEL I 3 sets **LEVEL II** 5 sets **LEVEL III** 7 sets **REST** up to 2 minutes

10 squats

2 plank walk-outs

10 shoulder taps

10 squats

2 plank walk-outs

10 plank rotations

10 squats

2 plank walk-outs

10-count plank hold

#22

NOTES

date

_____

total time

_____

set counter

☐ ☐ ☐ ☐ ☐ ☐ ☐

THE CRUSHER

DAREBEE WORKOUT © darebee.com

LEVEL I 3 sets **LEVEL II** 5 sets **LEVEL III** 7 sets **REST** up to 2 minutes

5 jump squats

10 lunges

one tricep extension

5 jump squats

10 calf raises

one tricep extension

5 jump squats

10-count plank

one tricep extension

#23

NOTES

date

_____

total time

_____

set counter

□ □ □ □ □ □ □

Dragon Reborn

DAREBEE WORKOUT © darebee.com

LEVEL I 3 sets **LEVEL II** 5 sets **LEVEL III** 7 sets **REST** up to 2 minutes

10 squats

4 side-to-side lunges

10 squats

4 dragon push-ups

2 plank walk-outs

4 dragon push-ups

10 knee-in & twists

4 sit-ups

10 knee-in & twists

#24

NOTES

date

_____

total time

_____

set counter

☐ ☐ ☐ ☐ ☐ ☐ ☐

EASY
DOES IT

DAREBEE WORKOUT © darebee.com

LEVEL I 3 sets **LEVEL II** 5 sets **LEVEL III** 7 sets **REST** up to 2 minutes

10 step jacks

20 side leg raises

10 step jacks

20 raised arm circles

10 step jacks

20 raised arm circles

#25

NOTES

date

_____

total time

_____

set counter

☐ ☐ ☐ ☐ ☐ ☐ ☐

EVERYDAY HERO

DAREBEE
WORKOUT
© darebee.com
Level I   3 sets
Level II 5 sets
Level III 7 sets
2 minutes rest

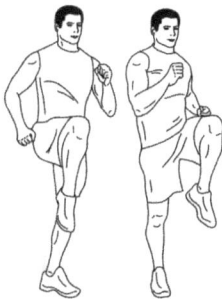

20 high knees

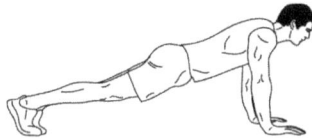

10-count plank hold

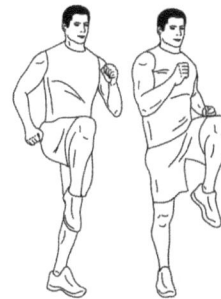

20 high knees

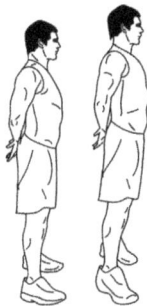

5 calf raises

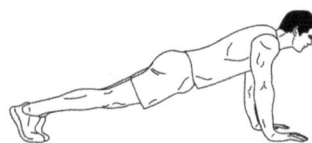

10-count plank hold

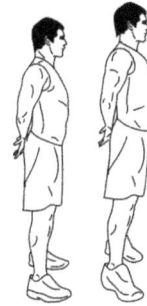

5 calf raises

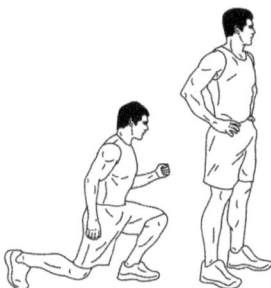

10 reverse lunges

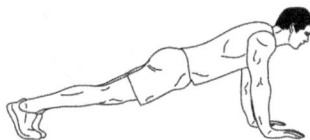

10-count plank hold

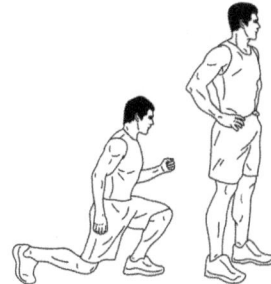

10 reverse lunges

#26

NOTES

date

_____

total time

_____

set counter

☐ ☐ ☐ ☐ ☐ ☐ ☐

EXPLORER

DAREBEE WORKOUT © darebee.com

LEVEL I 3 sets **LEVEL II** 5 sets **LEVEL III** 7 sets **REST** up to 2 minutes

20 march steps

10 shoulder taps

10 bicep extensions

20 march steps

10 scissor chops

10 arm scissors

20 march steps

10 chest expansions

10 raised arm circles

#27

NOTES

date

_____

total time

_____

set counter

☐ ☐ ☐ ☐ ☐ ☐ ☐

EXTRACTOR

DAREBEE WORKOUT © darebee.com

LEVEL I 3 sets **LEVEL II** 5 sets **LEVEL III** 7 sets **REST** up to 2 minutes

20 high knees

2 plank jump-ins

20 arm circles

20 half jacks

2 plank jump-ins

20 arm circles

2 jumping lunges

2 plank jump-ins

20 arm circles

#28
NOTES

date

_____

total time

_____

set counter

THE EXTRA MILE

DAREBEE WORKOUT
© darebee.com

Level I 3 sets
Level II 5 sets
Level III 7 sets
2 minutes rest

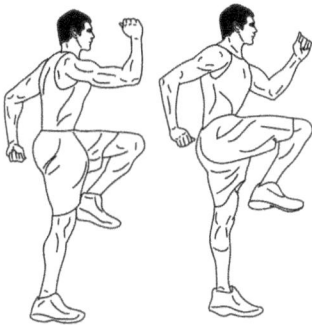

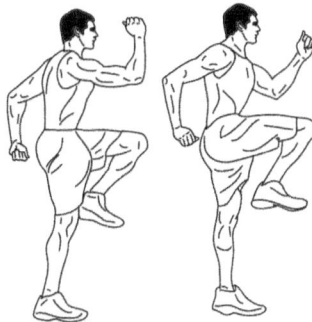

20 march steps

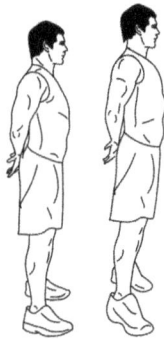

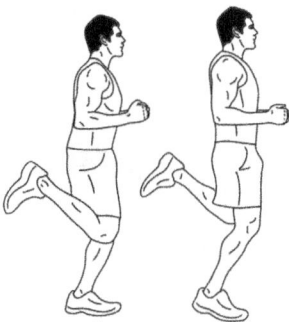

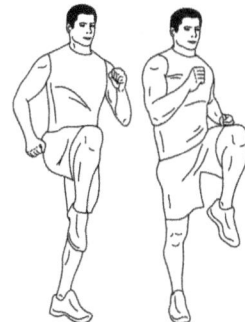

10 calf raises

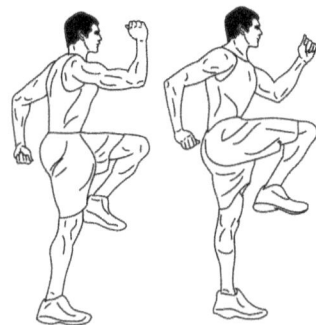

20 march steps

20 butt kicks

20 march steps

20 high knees

#29
NOTES

date

_____

total time

_____

set counter

☐ ☐ ☐ ☐ ☐ ☐ ☐

FALCON

DAREBEE WORKOUT © darebee.com

LEVEL I 3 sets **LEVEL II** 5 sets **LEVEL III** 7 sets **REST** up to 2 minutes

10 jumping jacks

6 plank rotations

6 plank crunches

10 jumping jacks

6 shoulder taps

6 plank jacks

10 jumping jacks

6 plank arm raises

6 slow climbers

#30

NOTES

date

_____

total time

_____

set counter

☐ ☐ ☐ ☐ ☐ ☐ ☐

the floor is
LAVA

DAREBEE WORKOUT © darebee.com

LEVEL I 3 sets **LEVEL II** 5 sets **LEVEL III** 7 sets **REST** up to 2 minutes

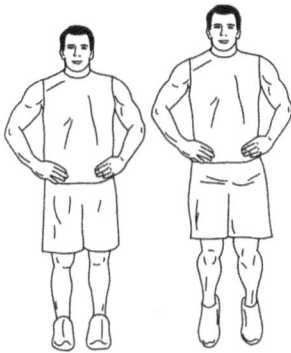

10 hops, feet together

10 jumping jacks

10 half jacks

10 jumping jacks

10 hops, feet apart

10 jumping jacks

#31
NOTES

date

_____

total time

_____

set counter

☐ ☐ ☐ ☐ ☐ ☐ ☐

FROST

DAREBEE WORKOUT © darebee.com

LEVEL I 3 sets **LEVEL II** 5 sets **LEVEL III** 7 sets **REST** up to 2 minutes

10 jumping jacks

10 arm circles

10 side leg raises

10 backward leg raises

10 twists

10 back kick + side leg raise

10 leg raises

10 flutter kicks

10 scissors

#32

NOTES

date

_____

total time

_____

set counter

☐ ☐ ☐ ☐ ☐ ☐ ☐

FUNDAMENTALS

DAREBEE WORKOUT © darebee.com

LEVEL I 3 sets **LEVEL II** 5 sets **LEVEL III** 7 sets **REST** up to 2 minutes

10 step jacks

10 march steps

10 single hip rotations

10 arm circles

10 chest expansions

10 bicep extensions

10 calf raises

10 side leg raises

10 side jacks

#33
NOTES

date

_____

total time

_____

set counter

☐ ☐ ☐ ☐ ☐ ☐ ☐

GAMBIT

DAREBEE WORKOUT © darebee.com

LEVEL I 3 sets **LEVEL II** 5 sets **LEVEL III** 7 sets **REST** up to 2 minutes

10 squats   **4** plank walk-outs   **10-count** plank hold

10 squats   **4** knee push-ups   **10-count** plank hold

10 squats   **4** plank-into-lunges   **10-count** plank hold

#34
NOTES

date

_____

total time

_____

set counter

☐ ☐ ☐ ☐ ☐ ☐ ☐

GOBLIN

DAREBEE WORKOUT © darebee.com

LEVEL I 3 sets **LEVEL II** 5 sets **LEVEL III** 7 sets **REST** up to 2 minutes

20 climbers

2 basic burpees with jump

20 climbers

10 get-ups

10 knee-ins with twist

10 get-ups

#35

NOTES

date

_____

total time

_____

set counter

☐ ☐ ☐ ☐ ☐ ☐ ☐

GOLEM

DAREBEE WORKOUT © darebee.com

LEVEL I 3 sets **LEVEL II** 5 sets **LEVEL III** 7 sets **REST** up to 2 minutes

10 lunges

4 jumping lunges

4 side lunges

4 push-ups

10 thigh taps

10-count plank

10 squats

10-count squat hold

4 jump squats

#36

NOTES

date

_____

total time

_____

set counter

☐ ☐ ☐ ☐ ☐ ☐ ☐

GRADE A

DAREBEE WORKOUT © darebee.com

LEVEL I 3 sets **LEVEL II** 5 sets **LEVEL III** 7 sets **REST** up to 2 minutes

10 cross squats

10 cossack squats

10 get-ups

5 judo push-ups

10-count push-up plank

10 up & down planks

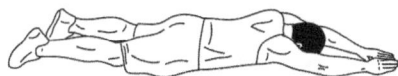

10 reverse angels

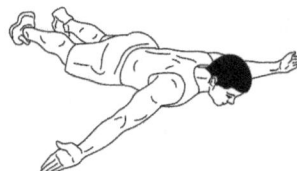

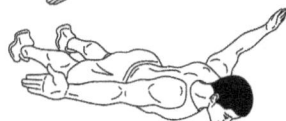

10 prone fly extensions

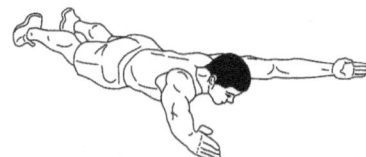

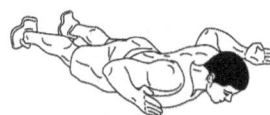

10 W-extensions

#37

NOTES

date

_____

total time

_____

set counter

☐ ☐ ☐ ☐ ☐ ☐ ☐

GRAVITY

DAREBEE WORKOUT © darebee.com

LEVEL I 3 sets **LEVEL II** 5 sets **LEVEL III** 7 sets **REST** 2 minutes

4 push-ups   **4** wide grip   **2** close grip

4 push-ups   **4** shoulder taps   **2** staggered

4 push-ups   **4** raised leg   **2** stacked feet

#38

NOTES

date

_____

total time

_____

set counter

☐ ☐ ☐ ☐ ☐ ☐ ☐

GUARDIAN

DAREBEE WORKOUT © darebee.com

LEVEL I 3 sets **LEVEL II** 5 sets **LEVEL III** 7 sets **REST** up to 2 minutes

8 squats

20 side leg raises

8 lunges

2 close grip push-ups

8 push-ups

10-count elbow plank

8 sit-ups

8 butt-ups

8 full bridges

#39
NOTES

date

_____

total time

_____

set counter

☐ ☐ ☐ ☐ ☐ ☐ ☐

HALL OF FAME

DAREBEE WORKOUT © darebee.com

LEVEL I 3 sets **LEVEL II** 5 sets **LEVEL III** 7 sets **REST** up to 2 minutes

20 march steps

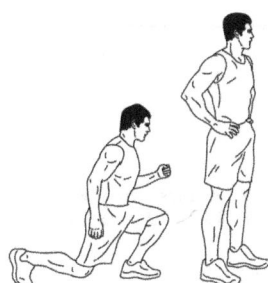

4 reverse lunges

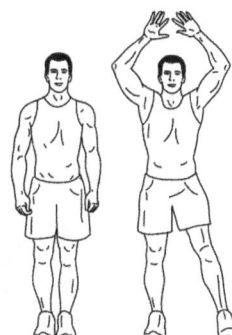

10 side leg raises

20 march steps

4 reverse lunges

10 bicep extensions

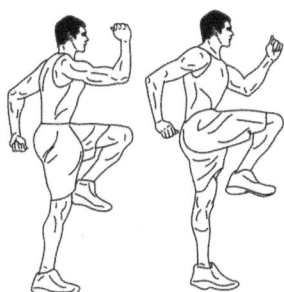

20 march steps

4 reverse lunges

10 step jacks

#40

NOTES

date

_____

total time

_____

set counter

☐ ☐ ☐ ☐ ☐ ☐ ☐

HERE & NOW

DAREBEE WORKOUT © darebee.com

LEVEL I 3 sets **LEVEL II** 5 sets **LEVEL III** 7 sets **REST** up to 2 minutes

20 march steps

6 reverse lunges

20 march steps

20-count stretch hold
right side

20 march steps

20-count stretch hold
left side

#41

NOTES

date

_____

total time

_____

set counter

☐ ☐ ☐ ☐ ☐ ☐ ☐

Hermit

DAREBEE WORKOUT © darebee.com

LEVEL I 3 sets **LEVEL II** 5 sets **LEVEL III** 7 sets **REST** up to 2 minutes

5 squats   **10-count** squat hold   **5** squats

5 knee push-ups   **10-count** knee push-up hold   **5** knee push-ups

5 crunches   **10-count** crunch hold   **5** crunches

#42
NOTES

date

_____

total time

_____

set counter

□ □ □ □ □ □ □

HERO

DAREBEE WORKOUT © darebee.com

LEVEL I 3 sets **LEVEL II** 5 sets **LEVEL III** 7 sets **REST** up to 2 minutes

10 squats

10-count squat hold

10 calf raises

5 push-ups

10-count plank hold

10 plank rotations

10 lunges

5 plank walk-outs

10 shoulder taps

#43

NOTES

date

_____

total time

_____

set counter

□ □ □ □ □ □ □

high burn

DAREBEE WORKOUT © darebee.com

LEVEL I 3 sets **LEVEL II** 5 sets **LEVEL III** 7 sets **REST** up to 2 minutes

10 jumping jacks

4 hop toe taps

10 jumping jacks

10 butt kicks

4 side-to-side jumps

10 butt kicks

10 half jacks

4 hop heel clicks

10 half jacks

#44

NOTES

date

_____

total time

_____

set counter

☐ ☐ ☐ ☐ ☐ ☐ ☐

HIT THE GROUND

DAREBEE
WORKOUT
© darebee.com
LEVEL I 3 sets
LEVEL II 5 sets
LEVEL III 7 sets
REST up to 2 minutes

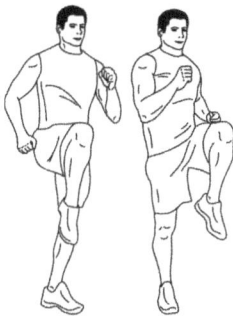

20 high knees

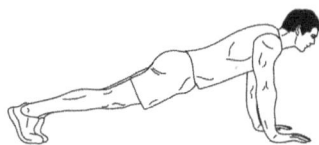

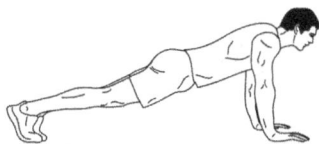

10-count plank hold

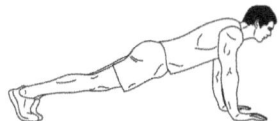

4 shoulder taps

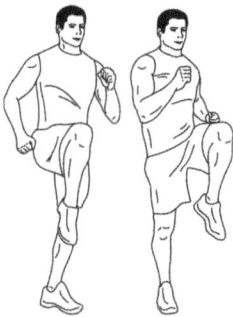

20 high knees

10-count plank hold

4 plank rotations

20 high knees

10-count plank hold

4 plank jacks

#45
NOTES

date

_____

total time

_____

set counter

☐ ☐ ☐ ☐ ☐ ☐ ☐

ICE AGE

DAREBEE WORKOUT © darebee.com

LEVEL I 3 sets **LEVEL II** 5 sets **LEVEL III** 7 sets **REST** up to 2 minutes

10 climbers **10** high knees **10** climbers

10 high knees **10** butt kicks **10** high knees

10 shoulder taps **10** high knees **10** shoulder taps

#46

NOTES

date

_____

total time

_____

set counter

☐ ☐ ☐ ☐ ☐ ☐ ☐

JOURNEYMAN

DAREBEE WORKOUT © darebee.com

LEVEL I 3 sets **LEVEL II** 5 sets **LEVEL III** 7 sets **REST** up to 2 minutes

10 reverse lunges

20 shoulder taps

10 plank rotations

10 reverse lunges

20 shoulder taps

10 climber taps

10 reverse lunges

20 shoulder taps

10 back extensions

#47

NOTES

date

_____

total time

_____

set counter

□ □ □ □ □ □ □

JOURNEY
BEFORE DESTINATION

DAREBEE WORKOUT © darebee.com

LEVEL I 3 sets **LEVEL II** 5 sets **LEVEL III** 7 sets **REST** up to 2 minutes

20 shoulder taps   **20** bicep extensions   **20** side shoulder taps

10 calf raises   **5** squats   **10** reverse lunges

10 side leg raises   **10** knee-to-elbows   **10** side bends

#48

NOTES

date

_____

total time

_____

set counter

☐ ☐ ☐ ☐ ☐ ☐ ☐

KINDER

DAREBEE WORKOUT © darebee.com

LEVEL I 3 sets **LEVEL II** 5 sets **LEVEL III** 7 sets **REST** up to 2 minutes

10 march steps

10 raised arm circles

10 march steps

10 arm extensions

10 march steps

10 bicep extensions

#49

NOTES

date

_____

total time

_____

set counter

☐ ☐ ☐ ☐ ☐ ☐ ☐

KNIGHT

DAREBEE WORKOUT © darebee.com

LEVEL I 3 sets **LEVEL II** 5 sets **LEVEL III** 7 sets **REST** up to 2 minutes

10 knight steps

10 side-to-side lunges   **10-count** squat hold   **10-count** folded squat hold

10 side shoulder taps   **10** shoulder taps   **10** elbow clicks

#50

NOTES

date

_____

total time

_____

set counter

☐ ☐ ☐ ☐ ☐ ☐ ☐

LAUNCHPAD

DAREBEE WORKOUT © darebee.com

LEVEL I 3 sets **LEVEL II** 5 sets **LEVEL III** 7 sets **REST** up to 2 minutes

10 butt kicks   **4** toe tap hops   **20** raised arm circles

10 butt kicks   **4** toe tap hops   **20** bicep extensions

10 butt kicks   **4** toe tap hops   **20** arm scissors

#51

NOTES

date

_____

total time

_____

set counter

☐ ☐ ☐ ☐ ☐ ☐ ☐

LAZY BEAR

DAREBEE WORKOUT © darebee.com

LEVEL I 3 sets **LEVEL II** 5 sets **LEVEL III** 7 sets **REST** up to 2 minutes

10 knee rolls

10 bridges

10 leg raises

10 W-extensions

10 reverse angels

#52

NOTES

date

_____

total time

_____

set counter

☐ ☐ ☐ ☐ ☐ ☐ ☐

LEVEL-UP!

DAREBEE WORKOUT © darebee.com

LEVEL I 3 sets **LEVEL II** 5 sets **LEVEL III** 7 sets **REST** up to 2 minutes

10 high knees

2 jumping lunges

10 bicep extensions

10 squats

2 jumping lunges

10 bicep extensions

#53
NOTES

date

_____

total time

_____

set counter

□ □ □ □ □ □ □

LIFEGUARD

DAREBEE WORKOUT © darebee.com

LEVEL I 3 sets **LEVEL II** 5 sets **LEVEL III** 7 sets **REST** up to 2 minutes

10 lunges

20 high knees

10 lunges

10 push-ups

20 high knees

10 push-ups

10 sit-ups

20 high knees

10 sit-ups

#54

NOTES

date

_____

total time

_____

set counter

☐ ☐ ☐ ☐ ☐ ☐ ☐

Low Impact

DAREBEE WORKOUT © darebee.com

LEVEL I 3 sets **LEVEL II** 5 sets **LEVEL III** 7 sets **REST** up to 2 minutes

20 march steps

10 calf raises

20 bicep extensions

20 alt arm/leg raises

20 leg extensions

20 side leg extensions

10 bridges

20 flutter kicks

10 dead bugs

#55

NOTES

date

_____

total time

_____

set counter

☐ ☐ ☐ ☐ ☐ ☐ ☐

MAGE

DAREBEE WORKOUT
© darebee.com

Level I 3 sets
Level II 5 sets
Level III 7 sets
2 minutes rest

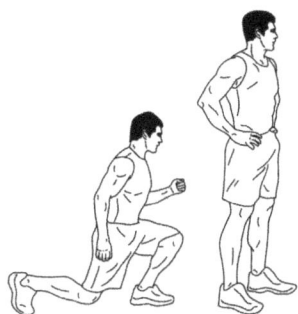

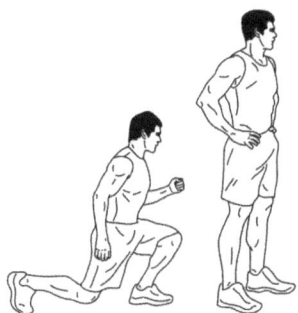

10 reverse lunges

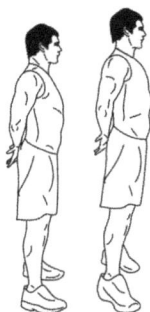

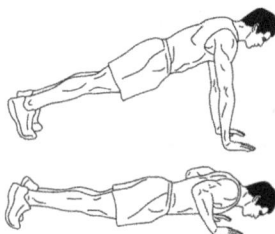

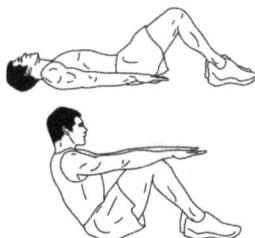

10 calf raises

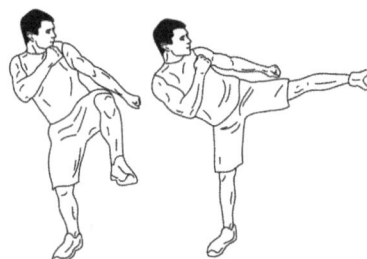

10 side kicks

10 reverse lunges

10 push-ups

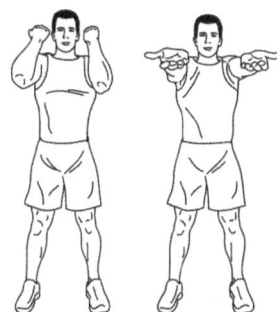

10 bicep extensions

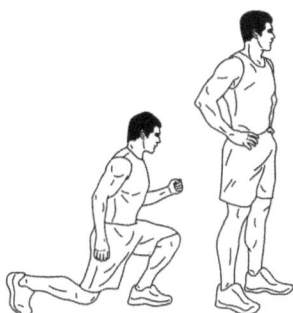

10 reverse lunges

10 sit-ups

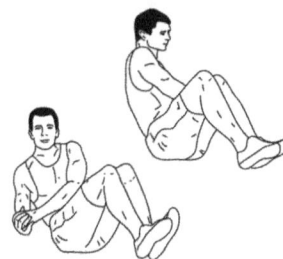

10 sitting twists

#56

NOTES

date

——————————

total time

——————————

set counter

☐ ☐ ☐ ☐ ☐ ☐ ☐

GO AHEAD
MAKE MY DAY

DAREBEE WORKOUT
© darebee.com
LEVEL I 3 sets
LEVEL II 5 sets
LEVEL III 7 sets
up to 2 minutes
rest between sets

2 push-ups

10 jumping jacks

2 push-ups

10 jumping lunges

2 push-ups

10 bicep extensions

#57
NOTES

date

_____

total time

_____

set counter

☐ ☐ ☐ ☐ ☐ ☐ ☐

MAVERICK

DAREBEE WORKOUT © darebee.com

LEVEL I 3 sets **LEVEL II** 5 sets **LEVEL III** 7 sets **REST** up to 2 minutes

10-count squat hold

5 jump squats

5 plank walk-outs

10 leg raises

5 raised leg circles

10 flutter kicks

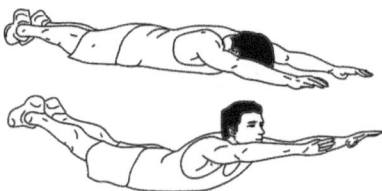

5 superman extensions

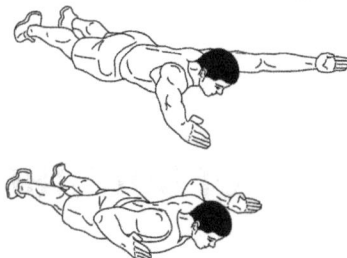

10 W-extensions

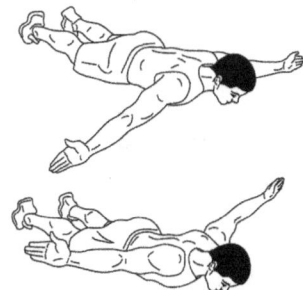

10 prone reverse fly

#58

NOTES

date

_____

total time

_____

set counter

☐ ☐ ☐ ☐ ☐ ☐ ☐

MEDIATOR

DAREBEE WORKOUT © darebee.com

LEVEL I 3 sets **LEVEL II** 5 sets **LEVEL III** 7 sets **REST** up to 2 minutes

20 shoulder taps

20 bicep extensions

20 shoulder taps

5 plank jacks

20 jumping jacks

5 plank jacks

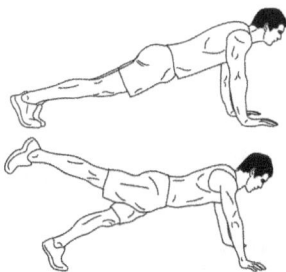

20 plank leg raises

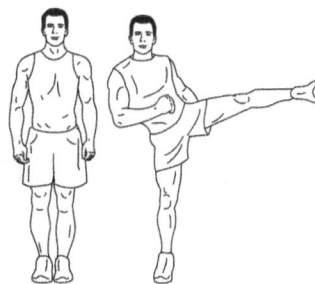

20 side leg raises

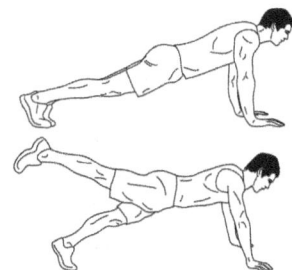

20 plank leg raises

#59
NOTES

date

_____

total time

_____

set counter

☐ ☐ ☐ ☐ ☐ ☐ ☐

YOU'VE GOT TO
MOVE IT MOVE IT'

WORKOUT
BY DAREBEE
© darebee.com

Level I 3 sets
Level II 5 sets
Level III 7 sets
2 minutes rest

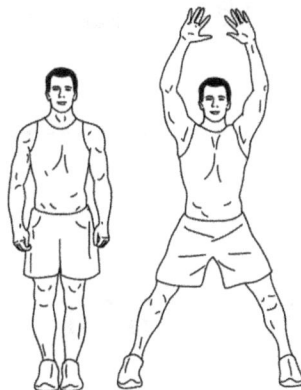

10 jumping jacks

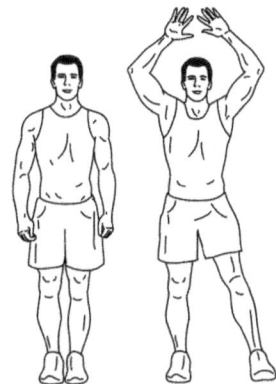

10 side jacks

10 jumping jacks

10 step jacks

10 jumping jacks

10 step jacks

#60

NOTES

date

_____

total time

_____

set counter

□ □ □ □ □ □ □

NEVER GIVE UP

DAREBEE WORKOUT © darebee.com

LEVEL I 3 sets **LEVEL II** 5 sets **LEVEL III** 7 sets **REST** up to 2 minutes

10 squats   **10-count** squat hold   **10** squats

10 shoulder taps   **10-count** plank hold   **10** shoulder taps

#61
NOTES

date

_____

total time

_____

set counter

☐ ☐ ☐ ☐ ☐ ☐ ☐

NEXT LEVEL

DAREBEE WORKOUT © darebee.com

LEVEL I 3 sets **LEVEL II** 5 sets **LEVEL III** 7 sets **REST** up to 2 minutes

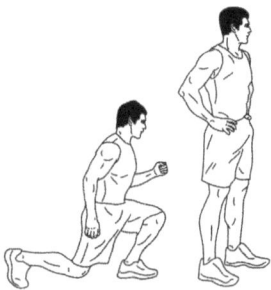

10 reverse lunges

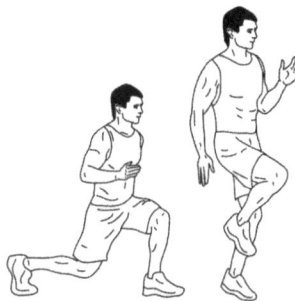

10 lunge step-ups

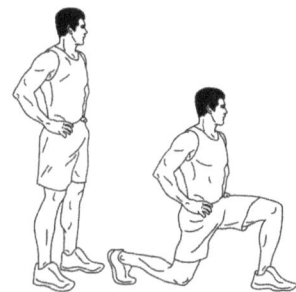

10 forward lunges

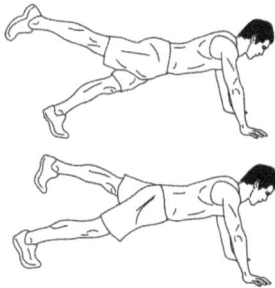

10 plank leg raises

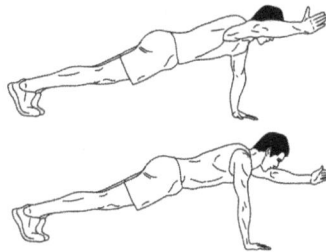

10 plank arm raises

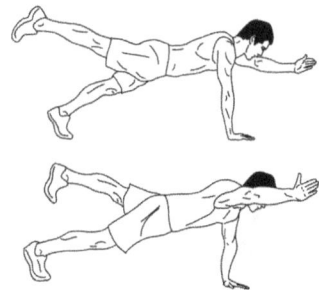

10 alt arm / leg raises

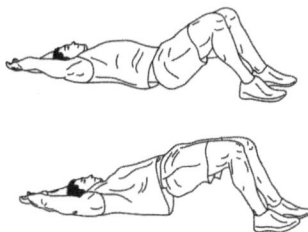

10 bridges

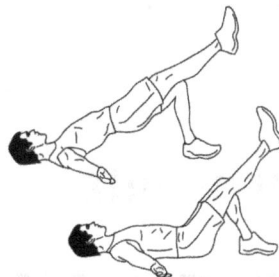

10 single leg bridges

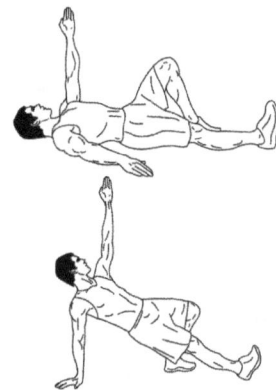

10 get-ups

#62

NOTES

date

_____

total time

_____

set counter

☐ ☐ ☐ ☐ ☐ ☐ ☐

NO CAPES

DAREBEE WORKOUT © darebee.com

LEVEL I 3 sets **LEVEL II** 5 sets **LEVEL III** 7 sets **REST** up to 2 minutes

10 squats

20 shoulder taps

10 squats

10-count plank

10-count raised leg plank

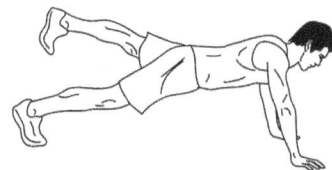

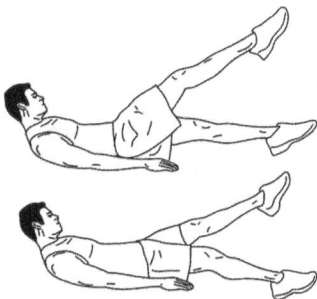

10-count raised leg plank

10 flutter kicks

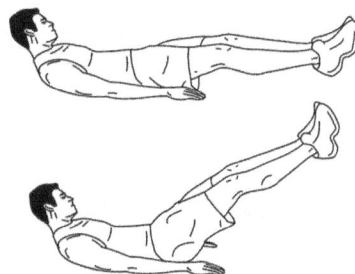

10 leg raises

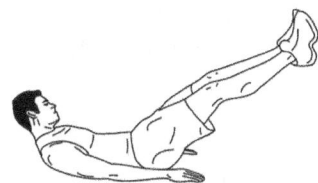

10-count raised legs hold

#63

NOTES

date

_____

total time

_____

set counter

☐ ☐ ☐ ☐ ☐ ☐ ☐

no-sweat
cardio

DAREBEE WORKOUT © darebee.com

LEVEL I 3 sets **LEVEL II** 5 sets **LEVEL III** 7 sets **REST** up to 2 minutes

10 step jacks

10 side step jacks

10 raised arm circles

10 march steps

10 step back + knee up

10 raised arm circles

10 side-to-side leg raises

10 side leg swings

10 raised arm circles

#64

NOTES

date

_____

total time

_____

set counter

☐ ☐ ☐ ☐ ☐ ☐ ☐

OVERLAP

DAREBEE WORKOUT © darebee.com

LEVEL I 3 sets **LEVEL II** 5 sets **LEVEL III** 7 sets **REST** up to 2 minutes

10 side bridges

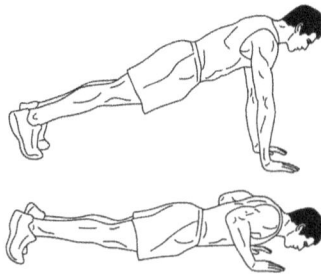

5 push-ups

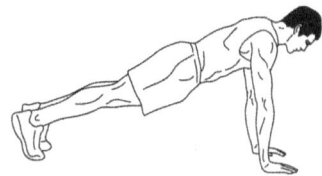

10-count plank hold

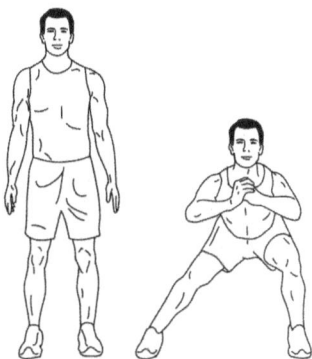

10 side lunges

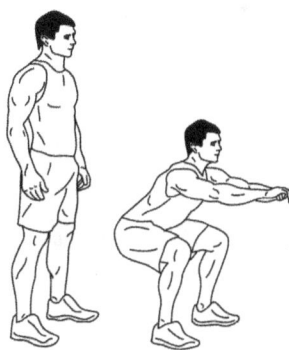

5 squats

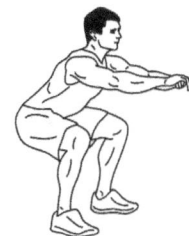

10-count squat hold

#65

NOTES

date

_____

total time

_____

set counter

☐ ☐ ☐ ☐ ☐ ☐ ☐

Perfect 10

DAREBEE WORKOUT © darebee.com

LEVEL I 3 sets **LEVEL II** 5 sets **LEVEL III** 7 sets **REST** up to 2 minutes

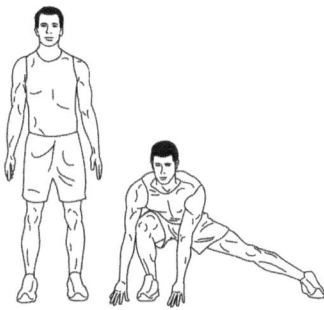

10 side lunges

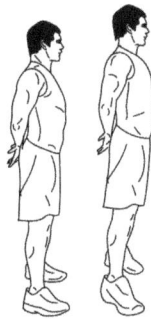

10 calf raises

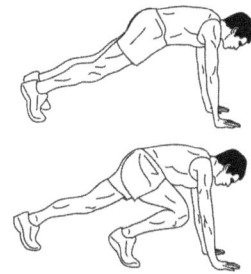

10 slow climbers

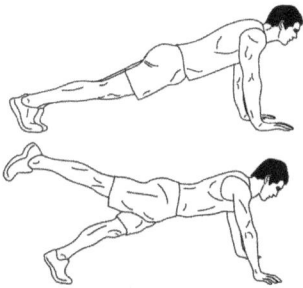

10 plank leg raises

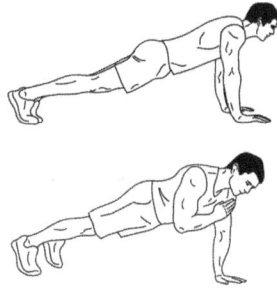

10 shoulder taps

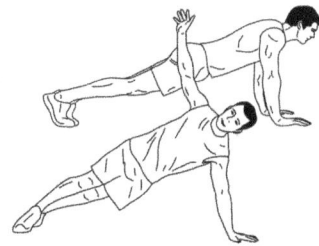

10 plank rotations

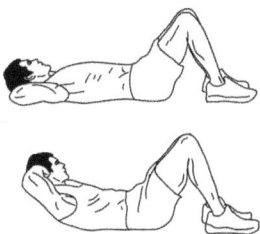

10 crunches

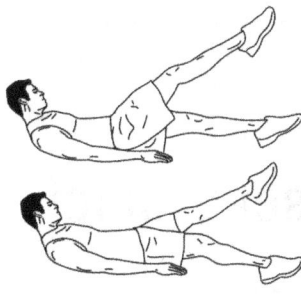

10 flutter kicks

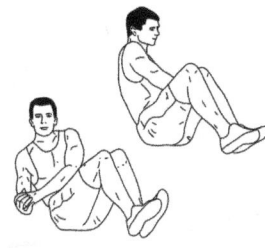

10 sitting twists

#66

NOTES

date

_____

total time

_____

set counter

☐ ☐ ☐ ☐ ☐ ☐ ☐

POWER CARDIO

DAREBEE WORKOUT
© darebee.com
LEVEL I 3 sets
LEVEL II 5 sets
LEVEL III 7 sets
REST up to 2 minutes

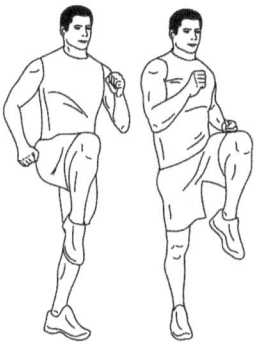

40 high knees

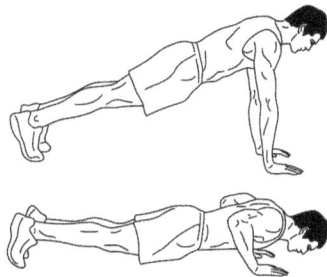

10 push-ups

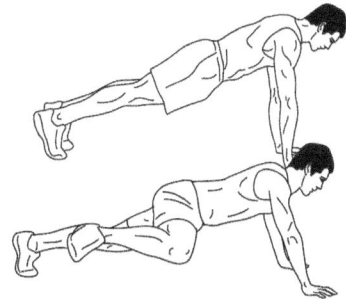

10 plank crunches

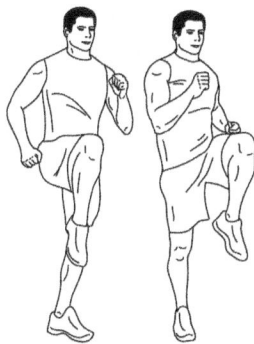

40 high knees

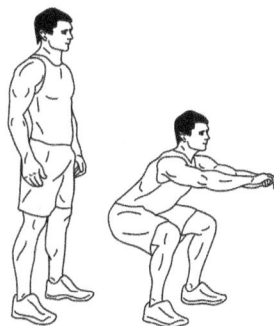

10 squats

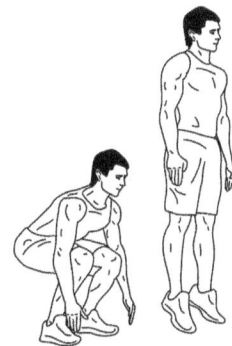

10 jump squats

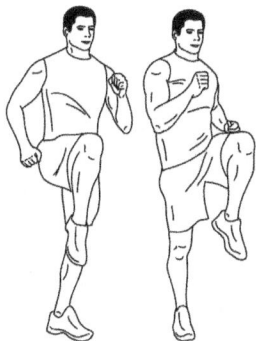

40 high knees

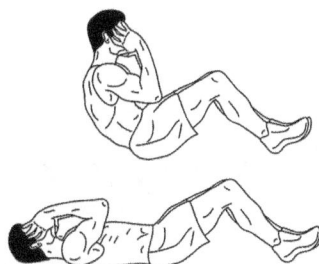

10 sit-ups

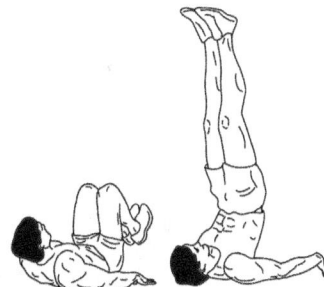

10 butt-ups

#67

NOTES

date

_____

total time

_____

set counter

☐ ☐ ☐ ☐ ☐ ☐ ☐

POWER CIRCUIT

DAREBEE WORKOUT © darebee.com

LEVEL I 3 sets **LEVEL II** 5 sets **LEVEL III** 7 sets **REST** up to 2 minutes

10 jump squats

10 push-ups

10 jumping lunges

30 bicep extensions

30sec elbow plank

30sec side elbow plank

#68

NOTES

date

_____

total time

_____

set counter

☐ ☐ ☐ ☐ ☐ ☐ ☐

power run

DAREBEE WORKOUT
© darebee.com

LEVEL I 3 sets **LEVEL II** 5 sets **LEVEL III** 7 sets **REST** up to 2 minutes

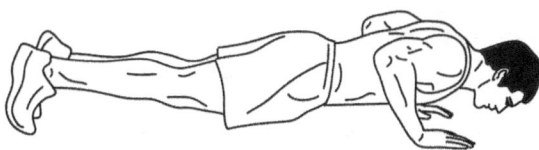

20 high knees

2 push-ups

20 high knees

2 push-ups

20 high knees

2 push-ups

20 high knees

2 push-ups

20 high knees

2 push-ups

20 high knees

2 push-ups

done

#69

NOTES

date

_____

total time

_____

set counter

☐ ☐ ☐ ☐ ☐ ☐ ☐

PROTAGONIST

DAREBEE WORKOUT © darebee.com

LEVEL I 3 sets **LEVEL II** 5 sets **LEVEL III** 7 sets **REST** up to 2 minutes

10 squats

5-count squat hold

10 side lunges

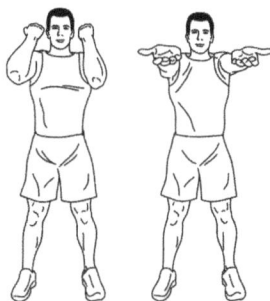

10 bicep extensions

10 arm circles

10 side shoulder taps

10 side leg raises

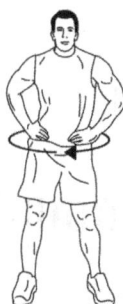

5 hip rotations

10 calf raises

#70

NOTES

date

_____

total time

_____

set counter

☐ ☐ ☐ ☐ ☐ ☐ ☐

PROTECTOR

DAREBEE WORKOUT © darebee.com

LEVEL I 3 sets **LEVEL II** 5 sets **LEVEL III** 7 sets **REST** up to 2 minutes

10 calf raises

20 squats

10 calf raises

20 scissor chops

20 arm scissors

20 scissor chops

10 bridges

10 leg raises

10 bridges

#71

NOTES

date

_____

total time

_____

set counter

□ □ □ □ □ □ □

PUSH-UP PARTY

DAREBEE WORKOUT © darebee.com

LEVEL I 3 sets **LEVEL II** 5 sets **LEVEL III** 7 sets **REST** up to 2 minutes

2 classic push-ups

2 raised leg push-ups

2 shoulder tap push-ups

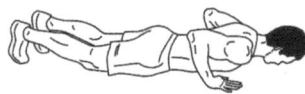

4 sky diver push-ups

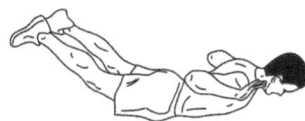

2 push-up side crunches

2 stacked push-ups

2 push-ups with rotation

#72

NOTES

date

_____

total time

_____

set counter

☐ ☐ ☐ ☐ ☐ ☐ ☐

RAW GRIT

DAREBEE WORKOUT © darebee.com

LEVEL I 3 sets **LEVEL II** 5 sets **LEVEL III** 7 sets **REST** up to 2 minutes

20 squats

20 push-ups

20 squats

20 calf raises

20 lunges

20 calf raises

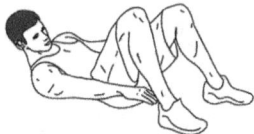

20 heel taps

20 crunches

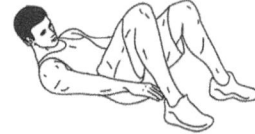

20 heel taps

#73

NOTES

date

_____

total time

_____

set counter

☐ ☐ ☐ ☐ ☐ ☐ ☐

REGENERATOR

DAREBEE WORKOUT © darebee.com

LEVEL I 3 sets **LEVEL II** 5 sets **LEVEL III** 7 sets **REST** up to 2 minutes

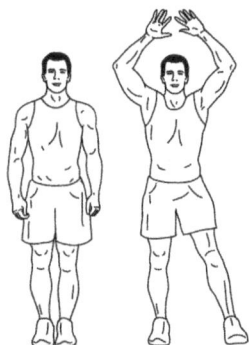

10 step jacks

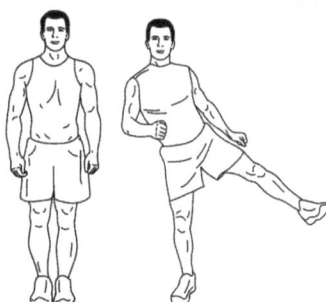

10 side leg raises

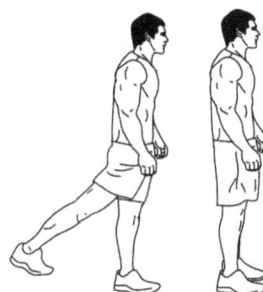

10 backward leg raises

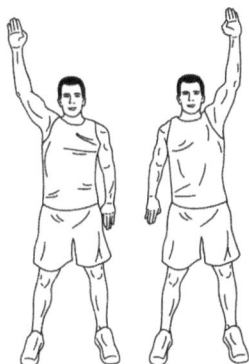

10 alt chest expansions

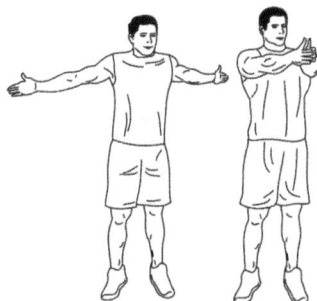

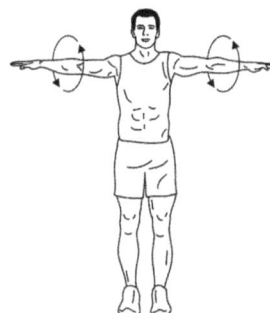

10 chest expansions

10 arm circles

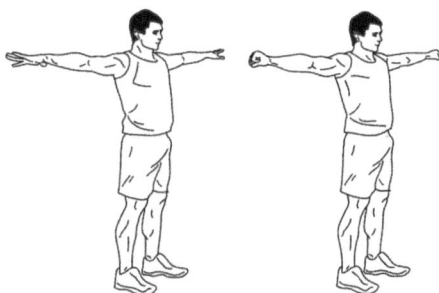

10 clench / unclench
arms to sides

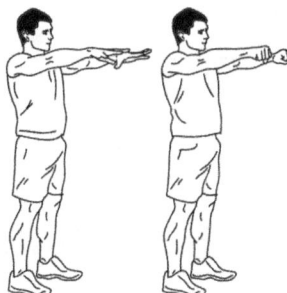

10 clench / unclench
arms forward

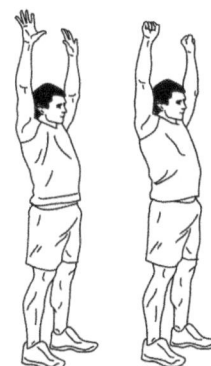

10 clench / unclench
arms overhead

#74
NOTES

date

_____

total time

_____

set counter

☐ ☐ ☐ ☐ ☐ ☐ ☐

THE ROASTER

DAREBEE WORKOUT © darebee.com

LEVEL I 3 sets **LEVEL II** 5 sets **LEVEL III** 7 sets **REST** up to 2 minutes

10 jumping jacks

one plank jack

one push-up

10 jumping jacks

one jump squat

one push-up

10 jumping jacks

two climber taps

one push-up

#75

NOTES

date

_____

total time

_____

set counter

☐ ☐ ☐ ☐ ☐ ☐ ☐

Rocking Around

DAREBEE WORKOUT © darebee.com

LEVEL I 3 sets **LEVEL II** 5 sets **LEVEL III** 7 sets **REST** up to 2 minutes

10 half jacks

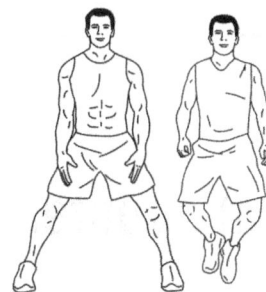

2 hop heel clicks

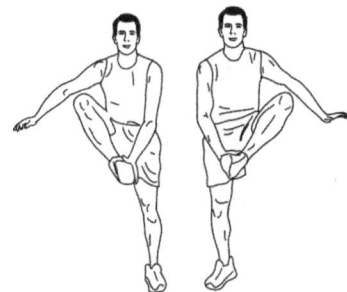

2 squats

10 half jacks

2 hop heel clicks

10 shoulder taps

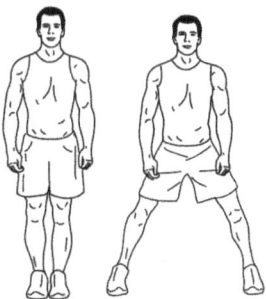

10 half jacks

2 hop heel clicks

2 hop heel taps

#76
NOTES

date

_____

total time

_____

set counter

☐ ☐ ☐ ☐ ☐ ☐ ☐

ROOKIE

DAREBEE WORKOUT © darebee.com

LEVEL I 3 sets **LEVEL II** 5 sets **LEVEL III** 7 sets **REST** up to 2 minutes

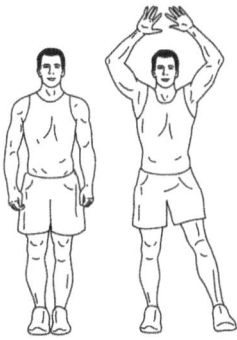

10 step jacks

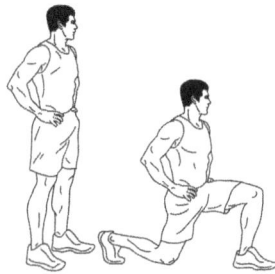

4 lunges

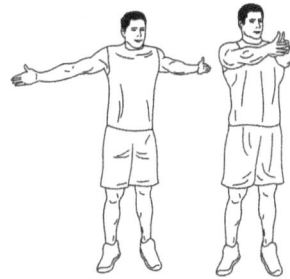

10 chest expansions

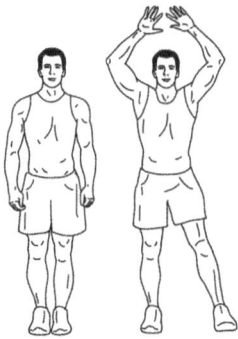

10 step jacks

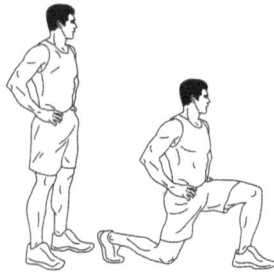

4 lunges

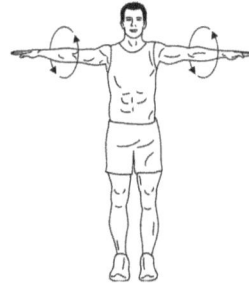

10 raised arm circles

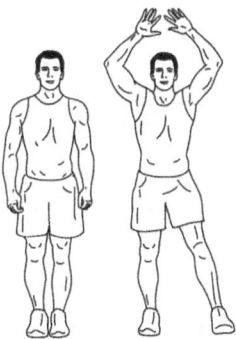

10 step jacks

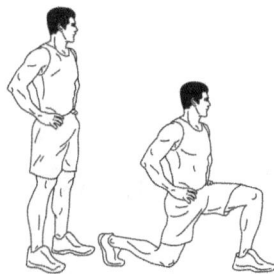

4 lunges

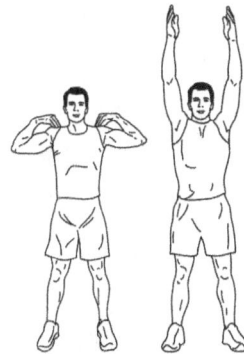

10 shoulder taps

#77

NOTES

date

_____

total time

_____

set counter

□ □ □ □ □ □ □

Roundabout

DAREBEE WORKOUT © darebee.com

LEVEL I 3 sets **LEVEL II** 5 sets **LEVEL III** 7 sets **REST** up to 2 minutes

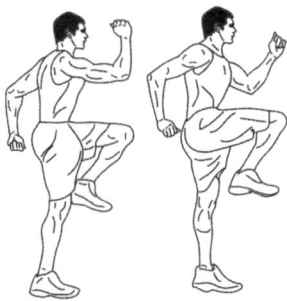

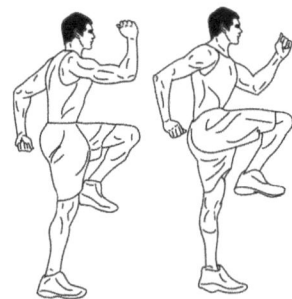

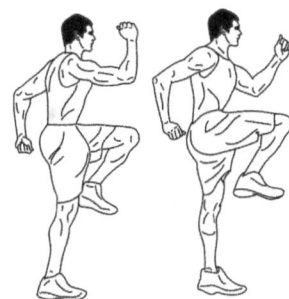

10 march steps

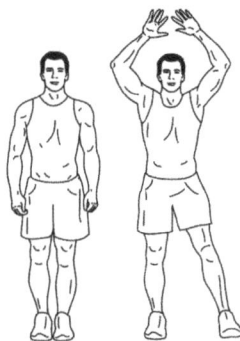

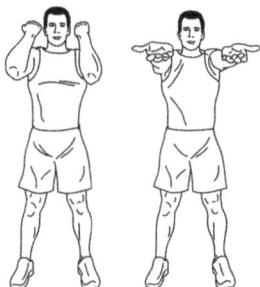

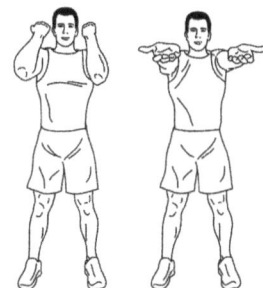

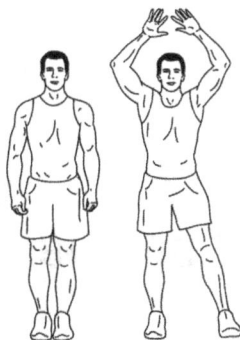

10 step jacks

10 march steps

10 bicep extensions

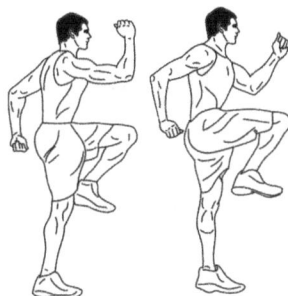

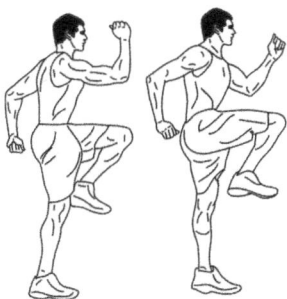

10 march steps

10 bicep extensions

10 march steps

10 step jacks

10 march steps

#78
NOTES

date

_____

total time

_____

set counter

☐ ☐ ☐ ☐ ☐ ☐ ☐

SAGE

DAREBEE WORKOUT © darebee.com

LEVEL I 3 sets **LEVEL II** 5 sets **LEVEL III** 7 sets **REST** up to 2 minutes

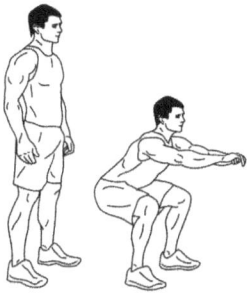

5 squats

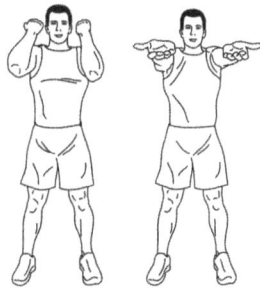

20 bicep extentions

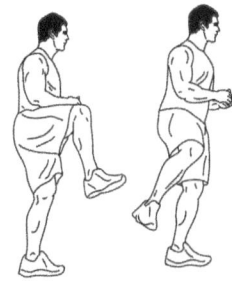

10 single hip rotations

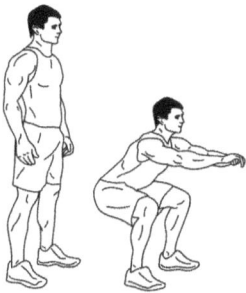

5 squats

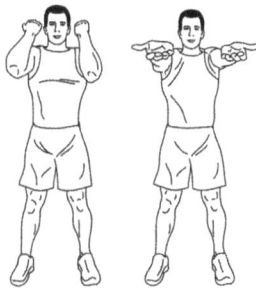

20 bicep extensions

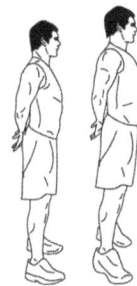

5 calf raises

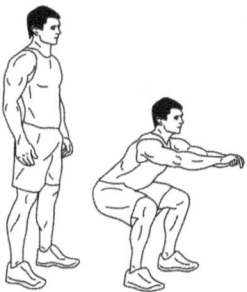

5 squats

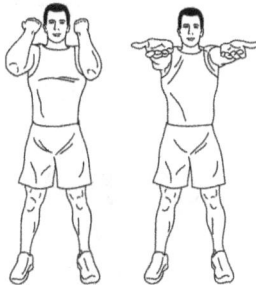

20 bicep extensions

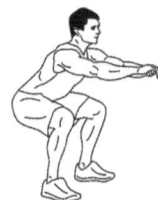

10-count squat hold

#79
NOTES

date

_____

total time

_____

set counter

☐ ☐ ☐ ☐ ☐ ☐ ☐

SHAPESHIFTER

DAREBEE WORKOUT © darebee.com

LEVEL I 3 sets **LEVEL II** 5 sets **LEVEL III** 7 sets **REST** up to 2 minutes

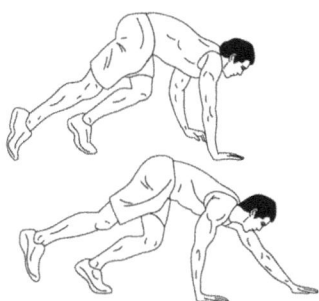

10-count bear crawl   **10** shoulder taps   **10** plank rotations

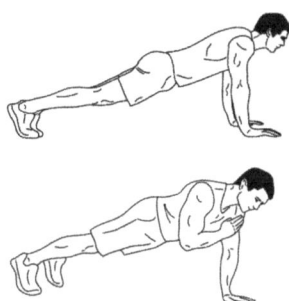

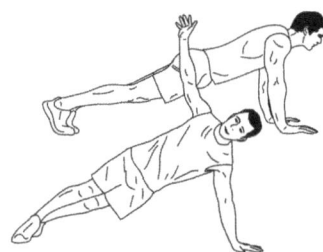

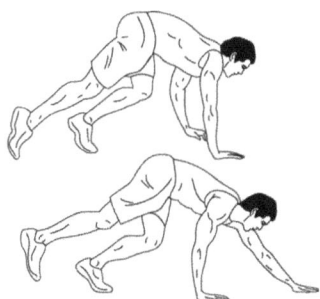

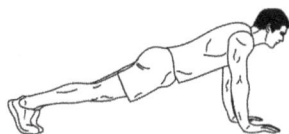

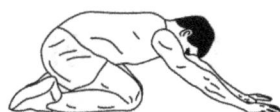

10-count bear crawl   **10-count** plank hold   **10** climber taps

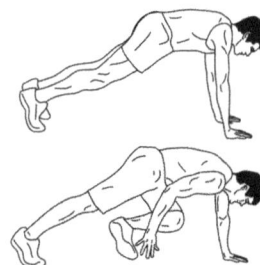

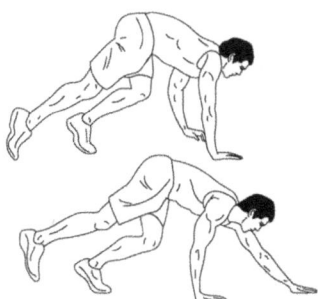

10-count bear crawl   **10-count** stretch #1   **10-count** stretch #2

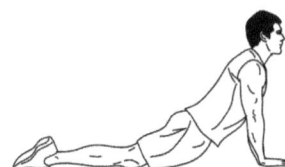

#80

NOTES

date

_____

total time

_____

set counter

☐ ☐ ☐ ☐ ☐ ☐ ☐

SO FAR
SO GOOD

DAREBEE WORKOUT © darebee.com

LEVEL I 3 sets **LEVEL II** 5 sets **LEVEL III** 7 sets **REST** up to 2 minutes

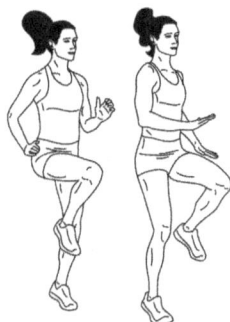

10 high knees

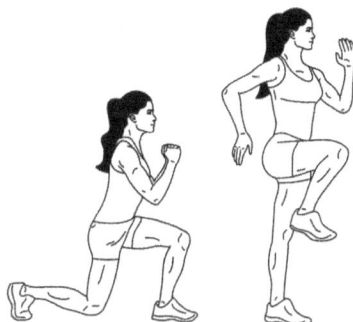

4 lunge step-ups

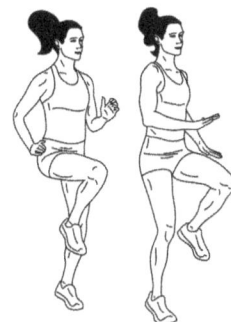

10 high knees

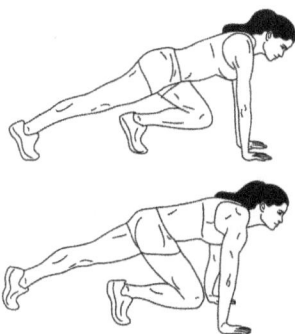

4 climbers

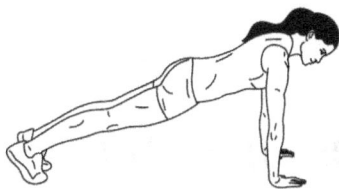

10-count plank hold

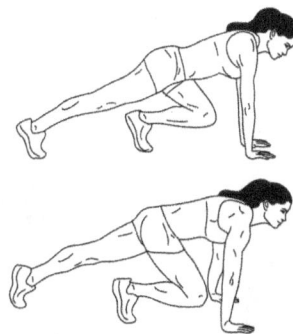

4 climbers

#81

NOTES

date

_____

total time

_____

set counter

☐ ☐ ☐ ☐ ☐ ☐ ☐

SPACEMAN

DAREBEE WORKOUT © darebee.com

LEVEL I 3 sets **LEVEL II** 5 sets **LEVEL III** 7 sets **REST** up to 2 minutes

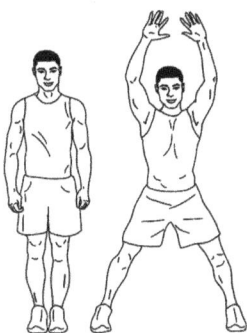

10 jumping jacks

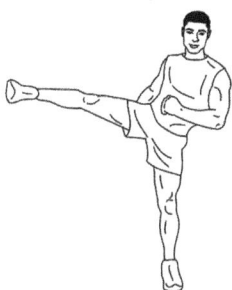

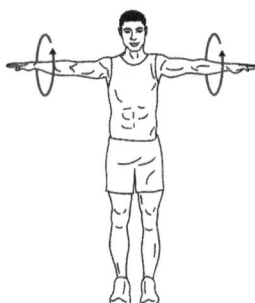

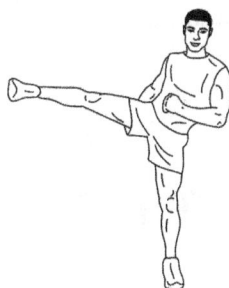

10-count right leg hold

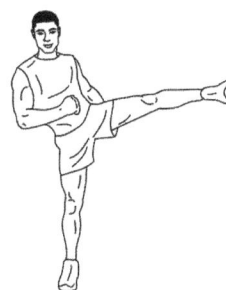

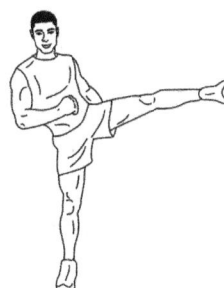

10-count left leg hold

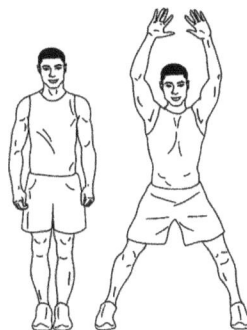

10 jumping jacks

20 raised arm circles

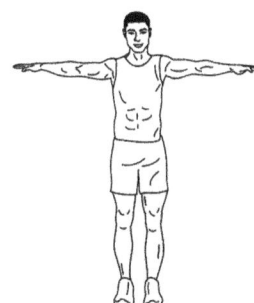

10-count arm hold

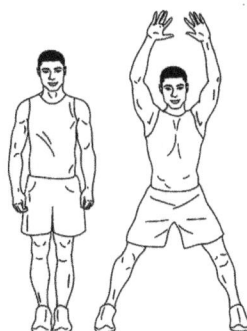

10 jumping jacks

10-count right leg hold

10-count left leg hold

#82

NOTES

date

_____

total time

_____

set counter

☐ ☐ ☐ ☐ ☐ ☐ ☐

SPARTAN

DAREBEE WORKOUT © darebee.com

LEVEL I 3 sets **LEVEL II** 5 sets **LEVEL III** 7 sets **REST** up to 2 minutes

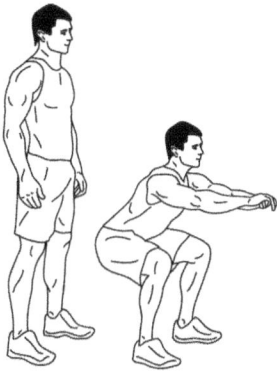

20 squats

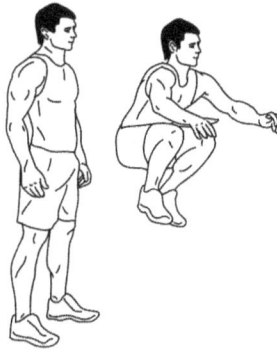

10 jump knee tucks

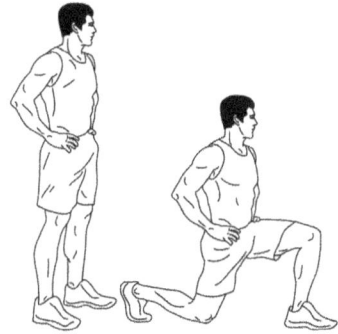

20 lunges

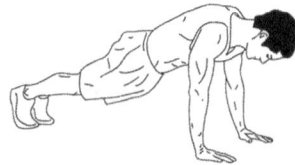

10 push-ups

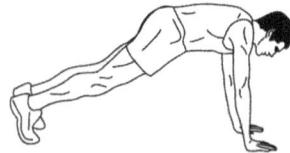
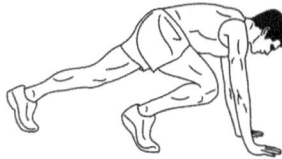

10 slow climbers

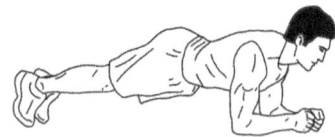

10-count elbow plank

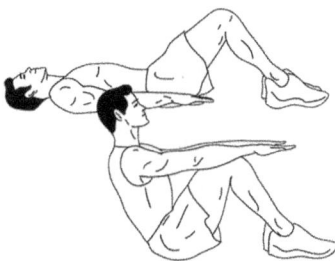

10 sit-ups

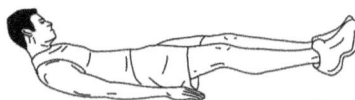
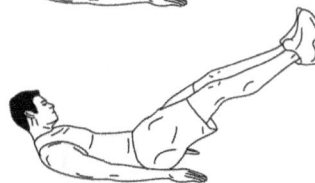

10 leg raises

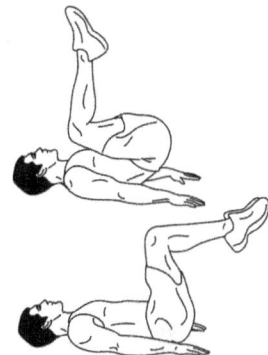

10 reverse crunches

#83

NOTES

date

_____

total time

_____

set counter

☐ ☐ ☐ ☐ ☐ ☐ ☐

STAND TALL

DAREBEE WORKOUT © darebee.com

LEVEL I 3 sets **LEVEL II** 5 sets **LEVEL III** 7 sets **REST** up to 2 minutes

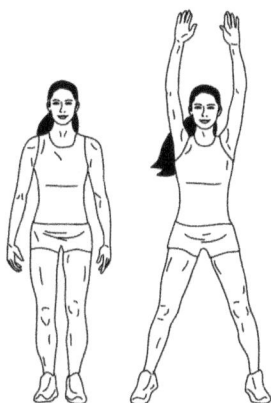

10 jumping jacks

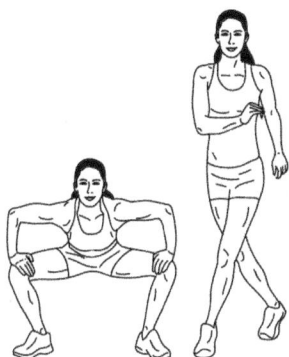

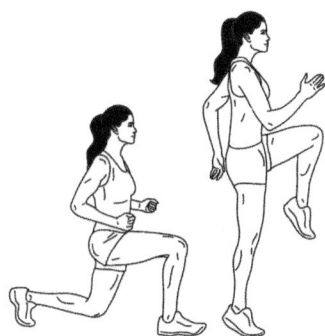

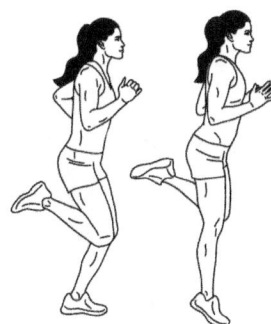

10 squat step back

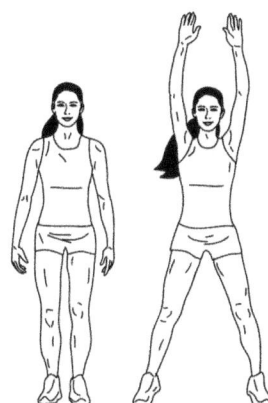

10 jumping jacks

10 lunge step-ups

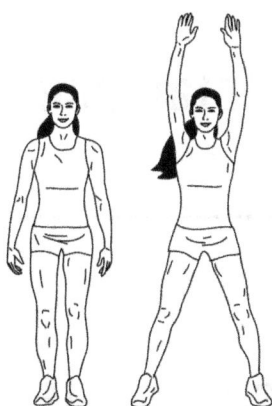

10 jumping jacks

10 butt kicks

#84

NOTES

date

_____

total time

_____

set counter

☐ ☐ ☐ ☐ ☐ ☐ ☐

STEP ONE

DAREBEE WORKOUT © darebee.com

LEVEL I 3 sets **LEVEL II** 5 sets **LEVEL III** 7 sets **REST** up to 2 minutes

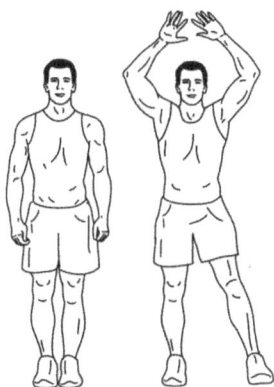

10 step jacks

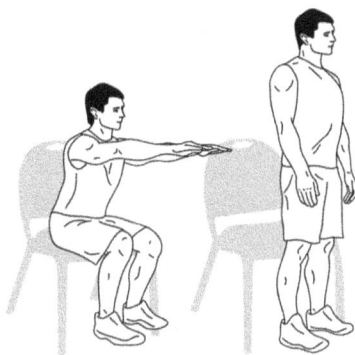

5 sit to stand

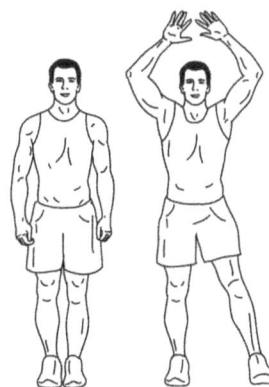

10 step jacks

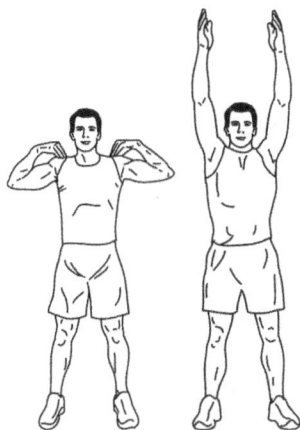

20 standing shoulder taps

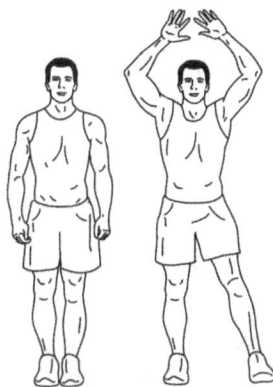

10 step jacks

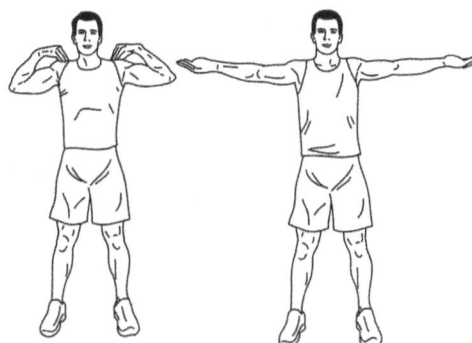

20 side bicep extensions

#85

NOTES

date

_____

total time

_____

set counter

☐ ☐ ☐ ☐ ☐ ☐ ☐

STOPGAP

DAREBEE WORKOUT © darebee.com

LEVEL I 3 sets **LEVEL II** 5 sets **LEVEL III** 7 sets **REST** up to 2 minutes

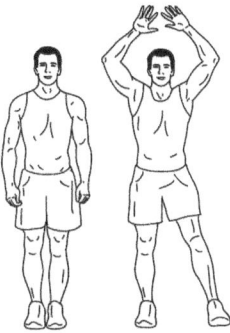

10 step jacks

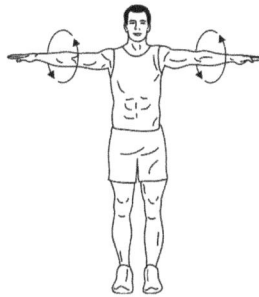

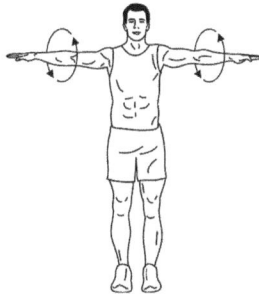

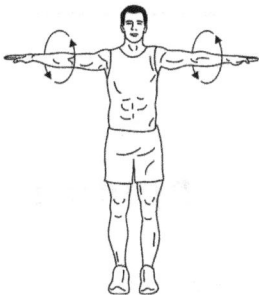

10 raised arm circles

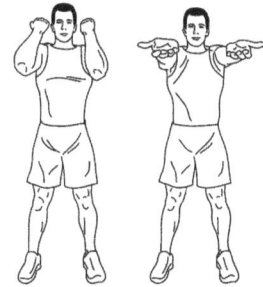

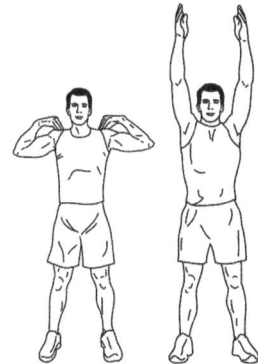

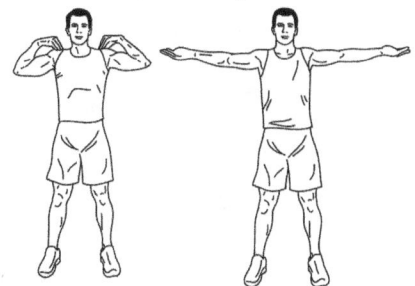

10 bicep extensions

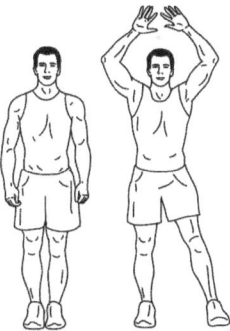

10 step jacks

10 raised arm circles

10 shoulder taps

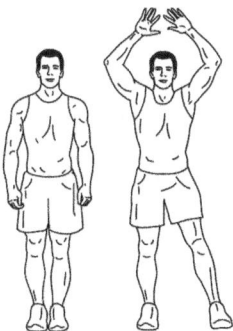

10 step jacks

10 raised arm circles

10 side shoulder taps

#86

NOTES

date

_____

total time

_____

set counter

□ □ □ □ □ □ □

STORY MODE

DAREBEE
WORKOUT
© darebee.com
Level I 3 sets
Level II 5 sets
Level III 7 sets
2 minutes rest

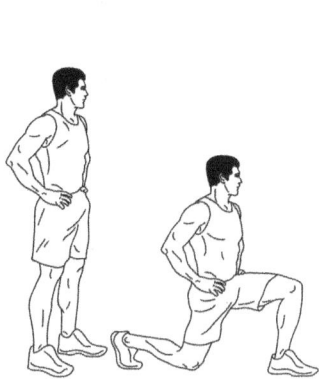

6 lunges

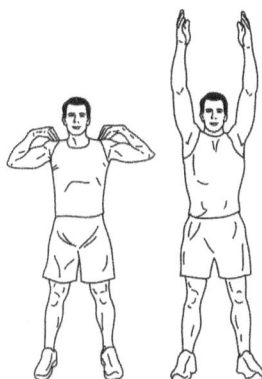

20 shoulder taps

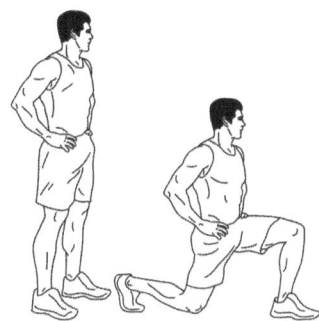

6 lunges

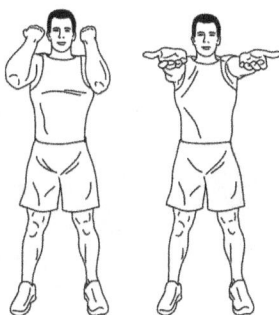

20 bicep extensions

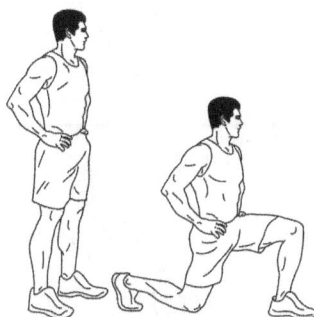

6 lunges

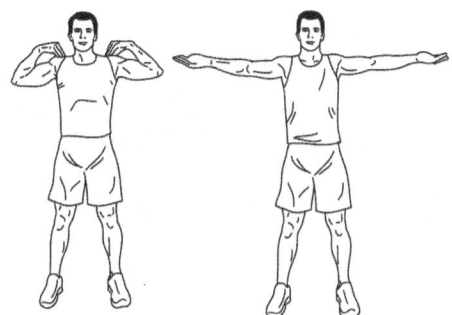

20 side shoulder taps

#87
NOTES

date

_____

total time

_____

set counter

☐ ☐ ☐ ☐ ☐ ☐ ☐

SUPER EASY

DAREBEE WORKOUT © darebee.com

LEVEL I 3 sets **LEVEL II** 5 sets **LEVEL III** 7 sets **REST** up to 2 minutes

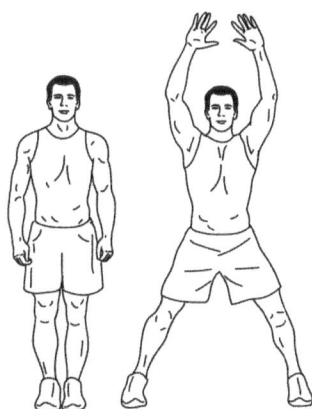

10 jumping jacks

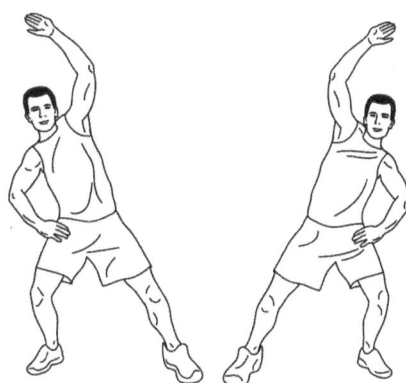

10 side jacks

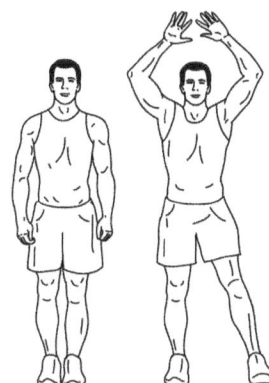

10 step jacks

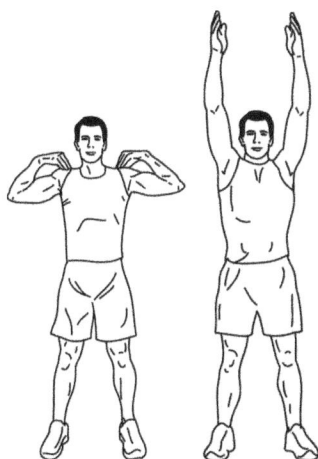

10 shoulder taps

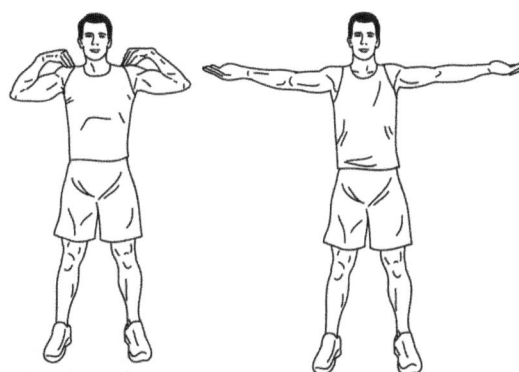

10 side shoulder taps

#88

NOTES

date

_____

total time

_____

set counter

☐ ☐ ☐ ☐ ☐ ☐ ☐

SUPERSTAR

DAREBEE WORKOUT © darebee.com

LEVEL I 3 sets **LEVEL II** 5 sets **LEVEL III** 7 sets **REST** up to 2 minutes

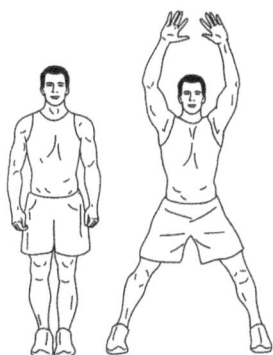

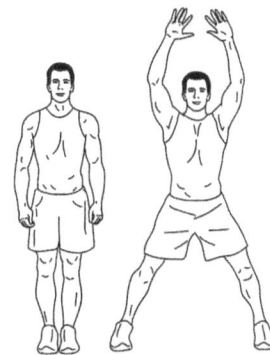

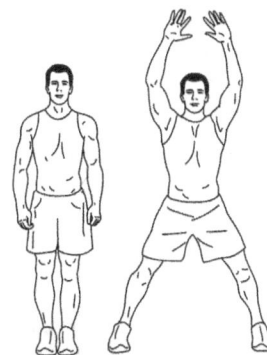

10 jumping jacks

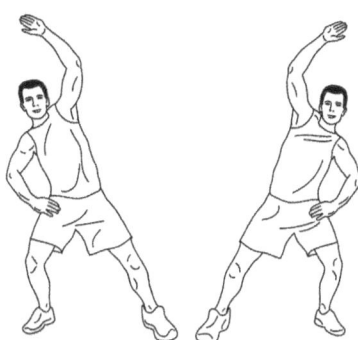

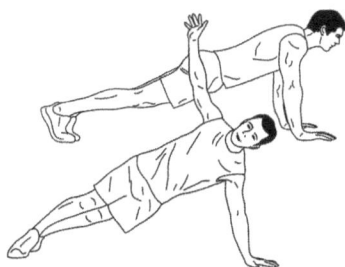

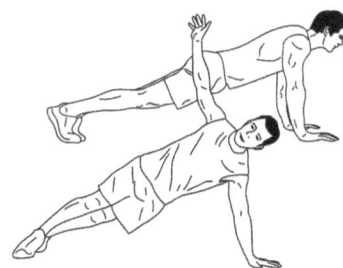

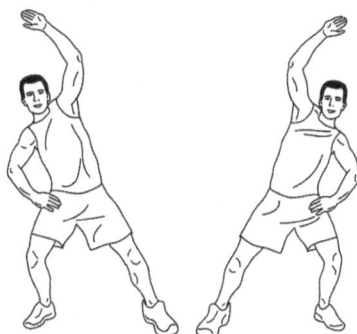

4 side jacks

10 jumping jacks

4 plank rotations

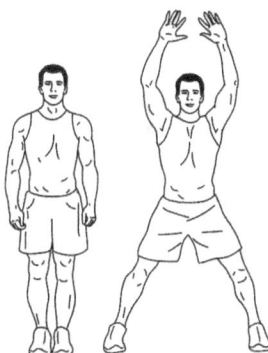

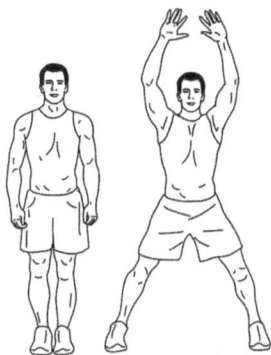

10 jumping jacks

4 plank rotations

10 jumping jacks

4 side jacks

10 jumping jacks

#89

NOTES

date

_____

total time

_____

set counter

☐ ☐ ☐ ☐ ☐ ☐ ☐

TEMPLE RUN

DAREBEE WORKOUT © darebee.com

LEVEL I 3 sets **LEVEL II** 5 sets **LEVEL III** 7 sets **REST** up to 2 minutes

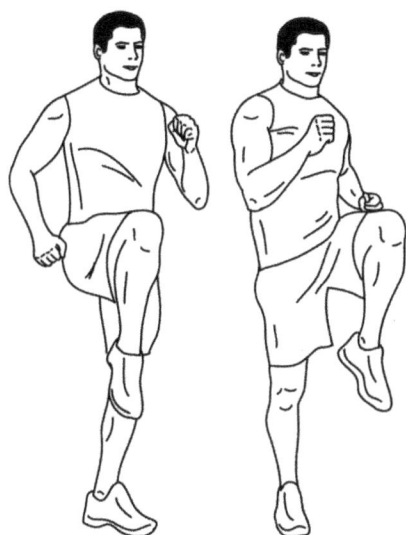

20 high knees

jump to the left

20 high knees

jump to the right

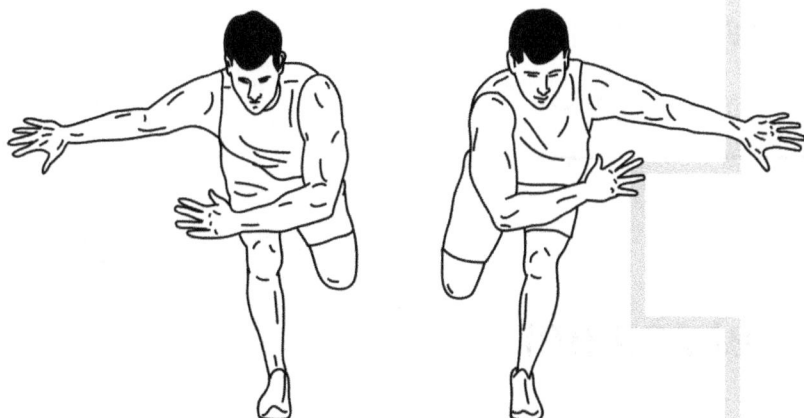

20 high knees

jump to the left

20 high knees

jump to the right

20 high knees

jump to the left

20 high knees

jump to the right

#90

NOTES

date

_____

total time

_____

set counter

☐ ☐ ☐ ☐ ☐ ☐ ☐

TOP *of the* WORLD

DAREBEE WORKOUT
© darebee.com

LEVEL I 3 sets
LEVEL II 5 sets
LEVEL III 7 sets
REST up to 2 minutes

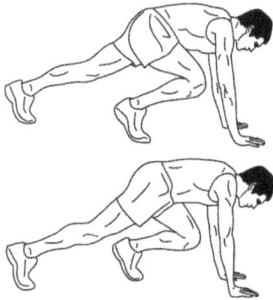

10 climbers

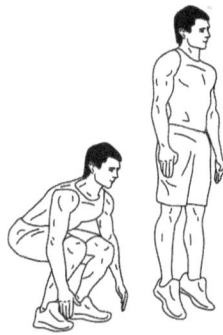

4 jump squats

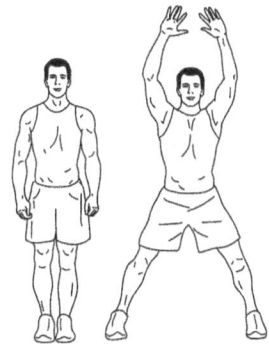

20 jumping jacks

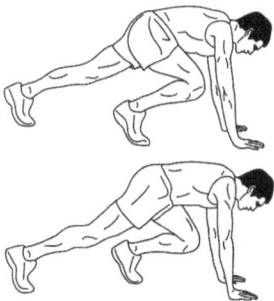

10 climbers

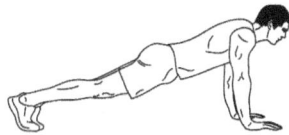

10-count plank hold

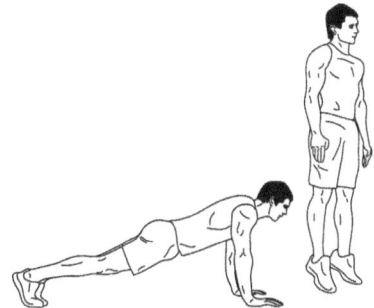

4 basic burpees

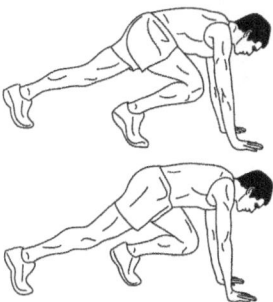

10 climbers

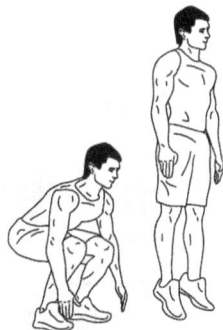

4 jump squats

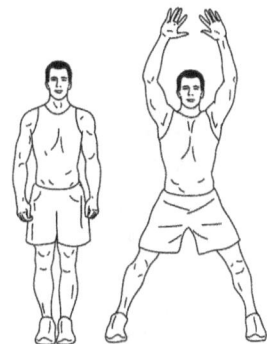

20 jumping jacks

#91
NOTES

date

_____

total time

_____

set counter

☐ ☐ ☐ ☐ ☐ ☐ ☐

Total Blast

DAREBEE WORKOUT © darebee.com

LEVEL I 3 sets **LEVEL II** 5 sets **LEVEL III** 7 sets **REST** up to 2 minutes

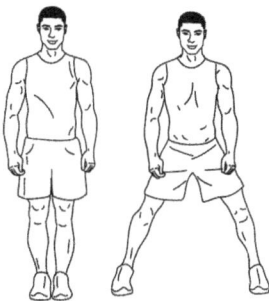

10 half jacks

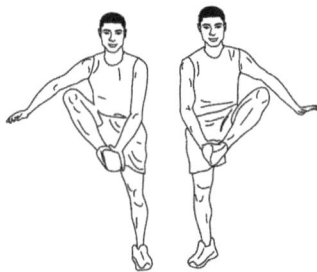

4 toe tap hops

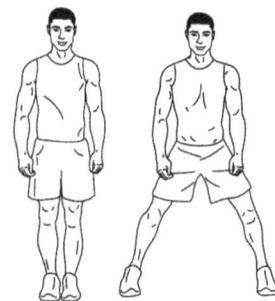

10 half jacks

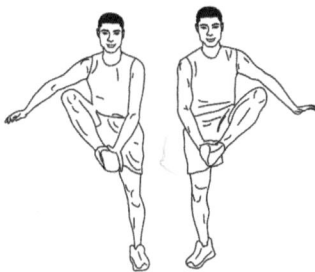

4 toe tap hops

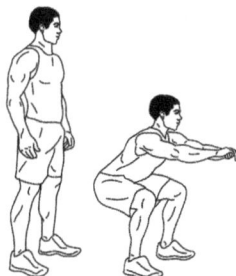

4 squats

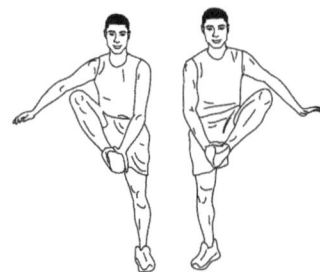

4 toe tap hops

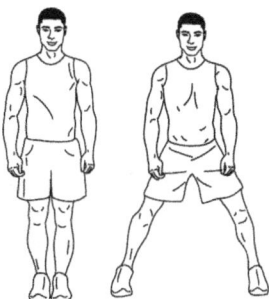

10 half jacks

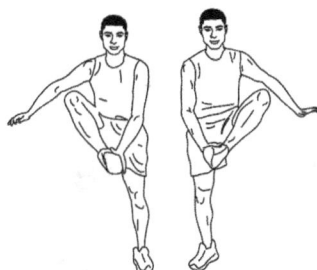

4 toe tap hops

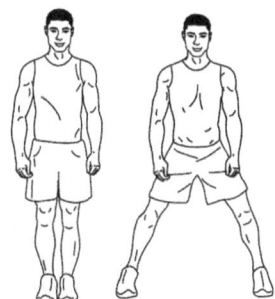

10 half jacks

#92

NOTES

date

——————————

total time

——————————

set counter

☐ ☐ ☐ ☐ ☐ ☐ ☐

TRACK&FIELD

DAREBEE WORKOUT © darebee.com

LEVEL I 3 sets **LEVEL II** 5 sets **LEVEL III** 7 sets **REST** up to 2 minutes

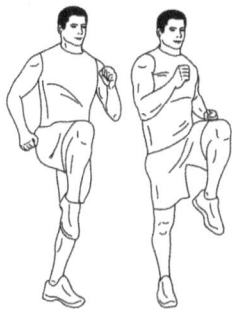

10 high knees

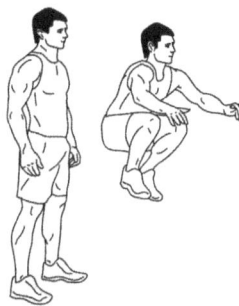

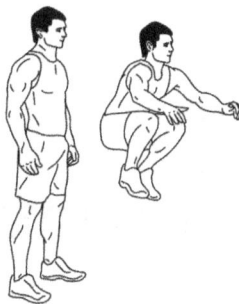

one jump knee tuck

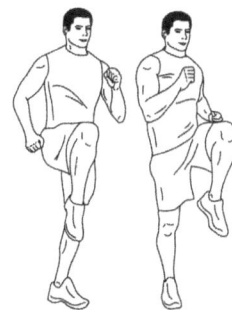

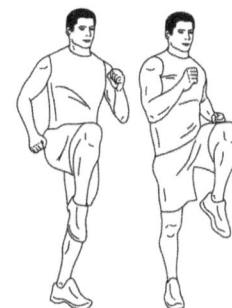

10 high knees

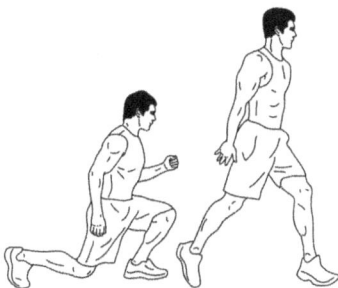

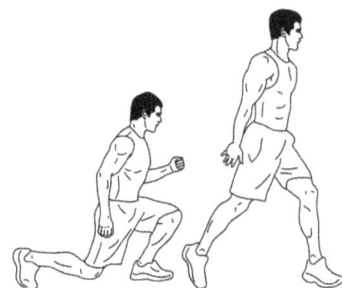

one jump lunge

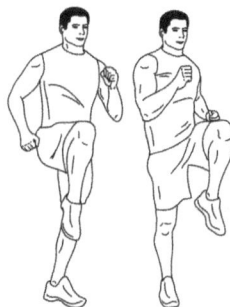

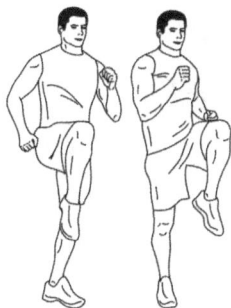

10 high knees

one jump lunge

10 high knees

one jump knee tuck

10 high knees

#93

NOTES

date

_____

total time

_____

set counter

☐ ☐ ☐ ☐ ☐ ☐ ☐

TRACKER

DAREBEE WORKOUT © darebee.com

LEVEL I 3 sets **LEVEL II** 5 sets **LEVEL III** 7 sets **REST** up to 2 minutes

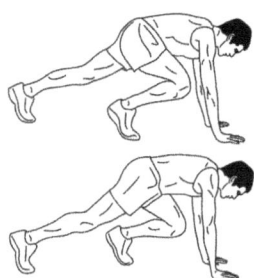

10 climbers

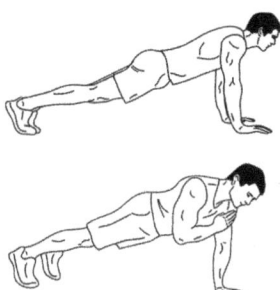

10 shoulder taps

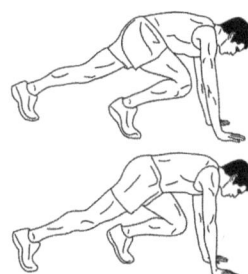

10 climbers

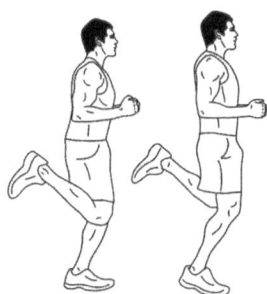

10 butt kicks

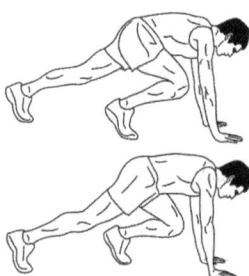

10 climbers

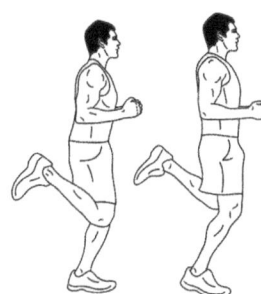

10 butt kicks

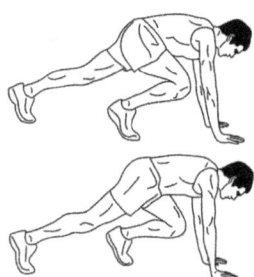

10 climbers

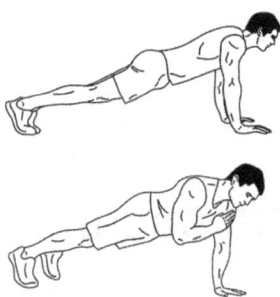

10 shoulder taps

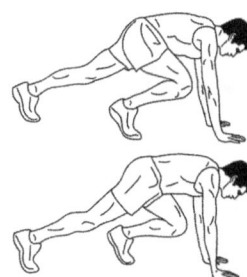

10 climbers

#94

NOTES

date

_____

total time

_____

set counter

☐ ☐ ☐ ☐ ☐ ☐ ☐

Triathlete

DAREBEE WORKOUT © darebee.com

LEVEL I 3 sets **LEVEL II** 5 sets **LEVEL III** 7 sets **REST** up to 2 minutes

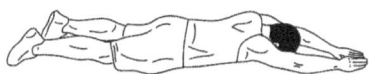

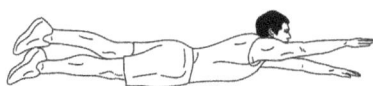

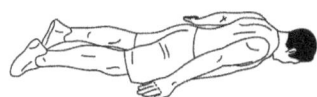

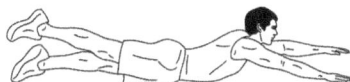

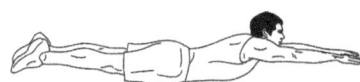

30 reverse angels

30 swim

10-count superman hold

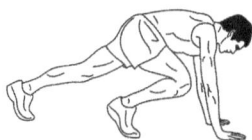

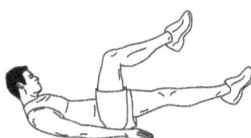

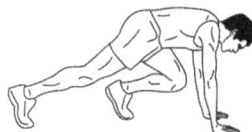

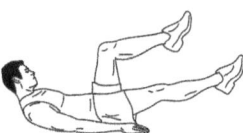

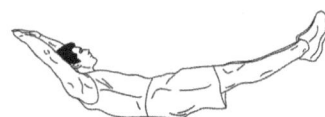

30 climbers

30 cycling crunches

10-count hollow hold

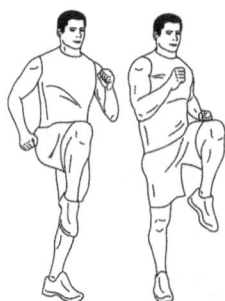

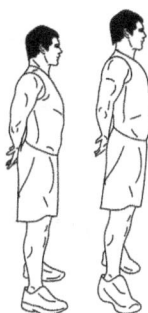

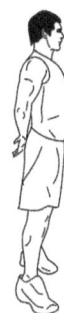

30 high knees

30 calf raises

10-count calf raise hold

#95

NOTES

date

_____

total time

_____

set counter

☐ ☐ ☐ ☐ ☐ ☐ ☐

Up & Down

DAREBEE WORKOUT © darebee.com

LEVEL I 3 sets **LEVEL II** 5 sets **LEVEL III** 7 sets **REST** up to 2 minutes

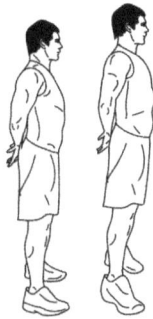
5 calf raises

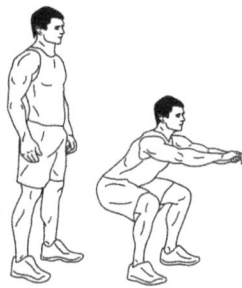
5 squats

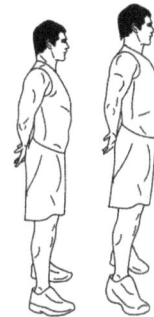
5 calf raises

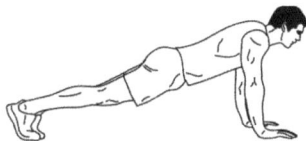
10-count plank hold

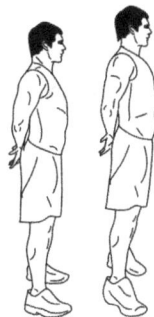
5 calf raises

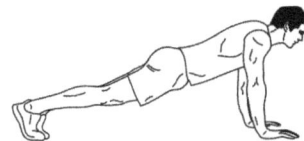
10-count plank hold

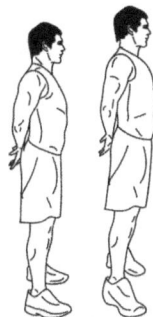
5 calf raises

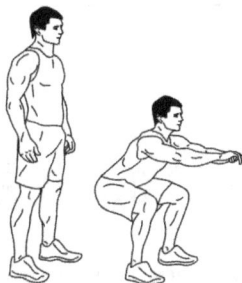
5 squats

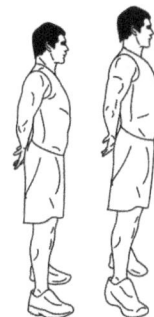
5 calf raises

#96

NOTES

date

_____

total time

_____

set counter

☐ ☐ ☐ ☐ ☐ ☐ ☐

THE UPGRADE

DAREBEE WORKOUT © darebee.com

LEVEL I 3 sets **LEVEL II** 5 sets **LEVEL III** 7 sets **REST** up to 2 minutes

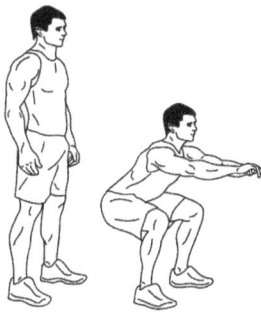

10 squats

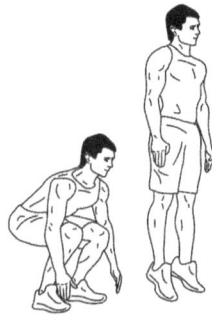

6 jump squats

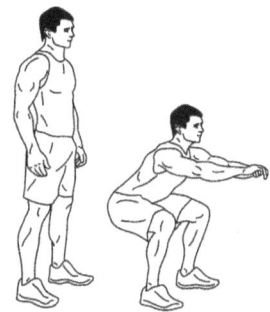

10 squats

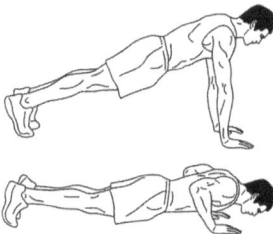

10 push-ups

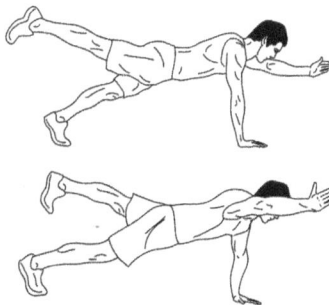

6 alt arm / leg raises

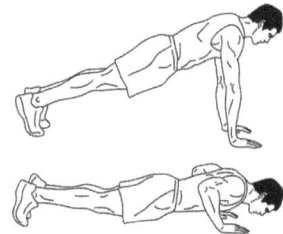

10 push-ups

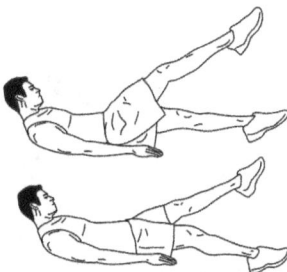

10 flutter kicks

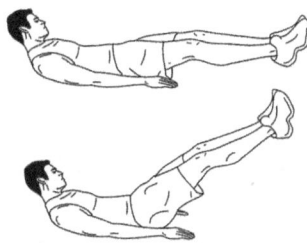

6 leg raises

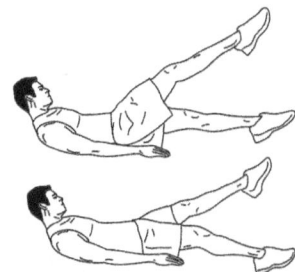

10 flutter kicks

#97
NOTES

date

_____

total time

_____

set counter

☐ ☐ ☐ ☐ ☐ ☐ ☐

UPPERBODY

DAREBEE WORKOUT © darebee.com

LEVEL I 3 sets **LEVEL II** 5 sets **LEVEL III** 7 sets **REST** up to 2 minutes

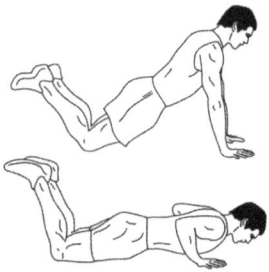

10 knee push-ups

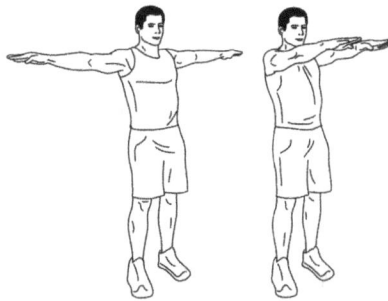

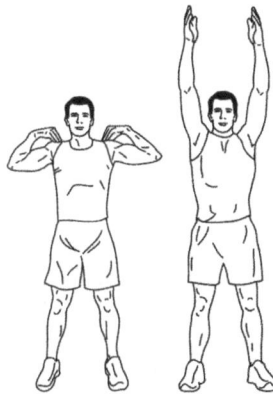

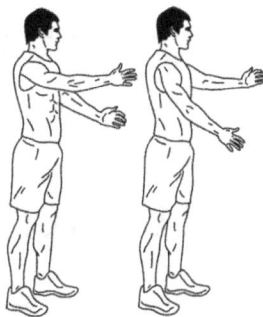

10 arm extensions

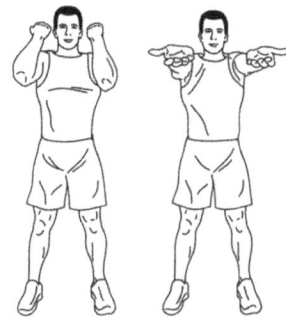

10 bicep extensions

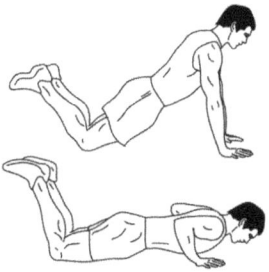

10 knee push-ups

10 shoulder taps

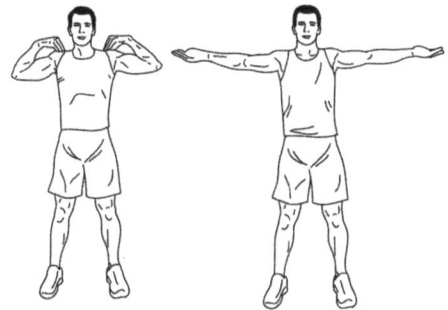

10 side shoulder taps

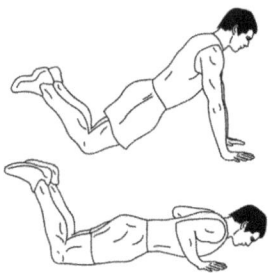

10 knee push-ups

10 scissor chops

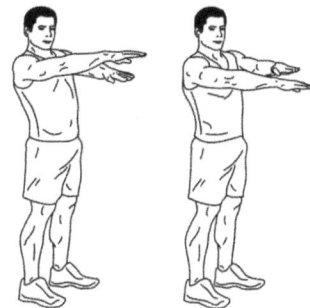

10 arm scissors

#98

NOTES

date

_____

total time

_____

set counter

☐ ☐ ☐ ☐ ☐ ☐ ☐

VICTORY LAP

DAREBEE WORKOUT
© darebee.com
LEVEL I 3 sets LEVEL II 5 sets LEVEL III 7 sets
up to 2 minutes rest between sets

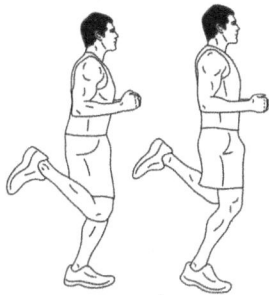

10 butt kicks

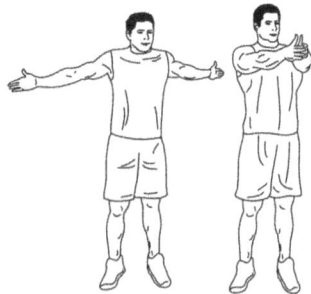

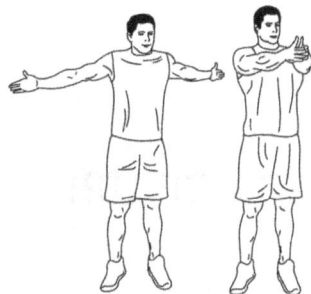

10 chest expansions

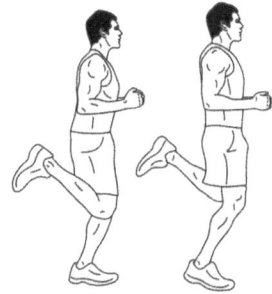

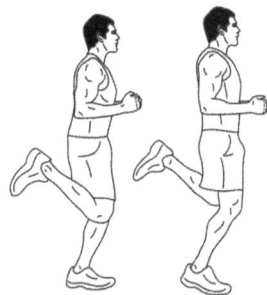

10 butt kicks

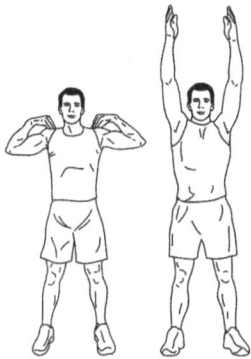

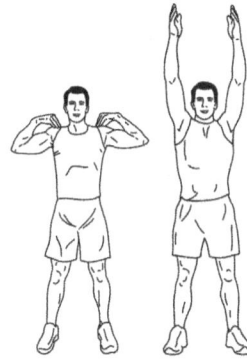

10 shoulder taps

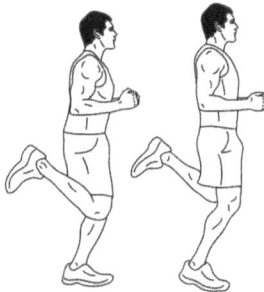

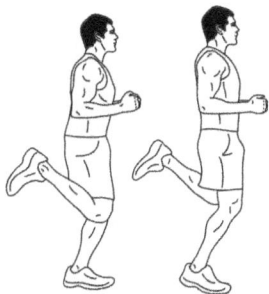

10 butt kicks

10 shoulder taps

10 butt kicks

10 chest expansions

10 butt kicks

#99

NOTES

date

_____

total time

_____

set counter

☐ ☐ ☐ ☐ ☐ ☐ ☐

WATCHMAN

DAREBEE WORKOUT © darebee.com

LEVEL I 3 sets **LEVEL II** 5 sets **LEVEL III** 7 sets **REST** up to 2 minutes

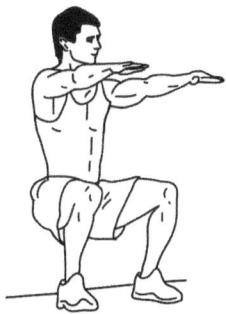

20sec wall-sit

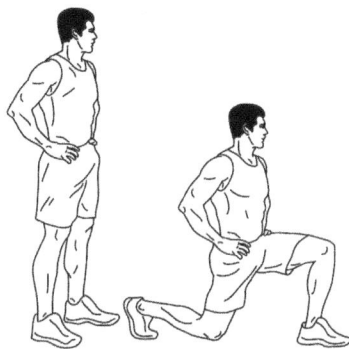

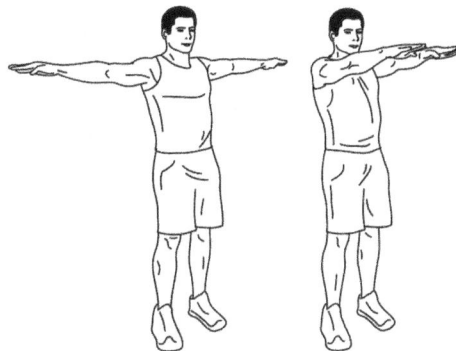

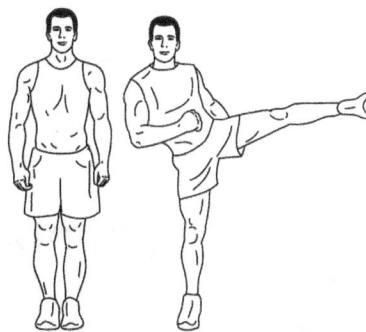

20 lunges

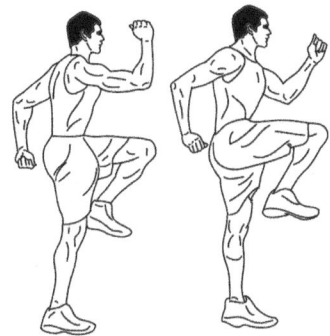

40 march steps

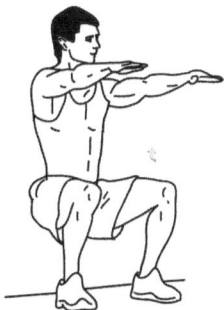

20sec wall-sit

40 arm extensions

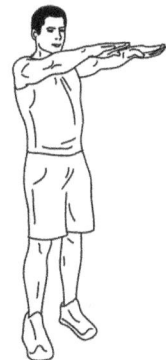

20sec raised arms hold

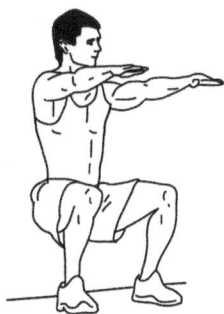

20sec wall-sit

40 side leg raises

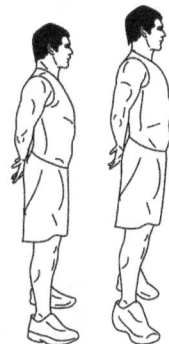

20 calf raises

#100

NOTES

date

_____

total time

_____

set counter

☐ ☐ ☐ ☐ ☐ ☐ ☐

white rabbit

DAREBEE WORKOUT © darebee.com

LEVEL I 3 sets **LEVEL II** 5 sets **LEVEL III** 7 sets **REST** up to 2 minutes

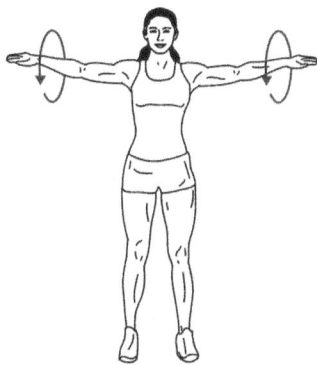

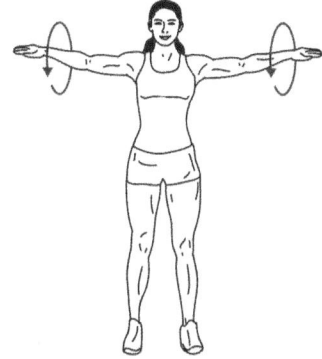

20 raised arm circles

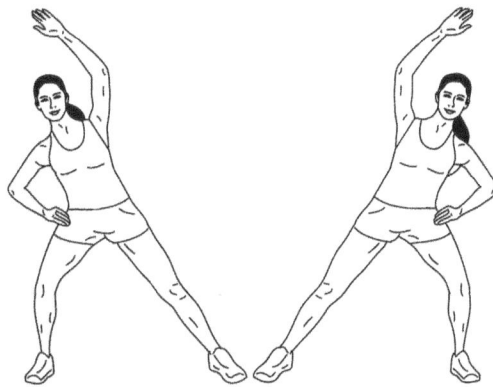

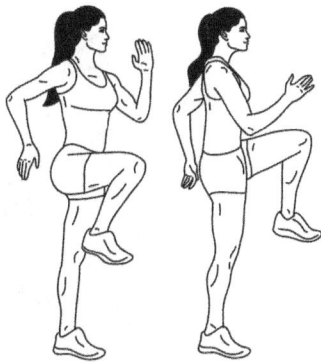

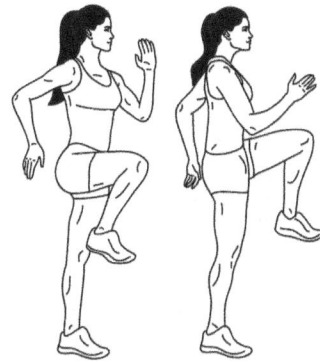

20 side jacks

20 raised arm circles

20 march steps

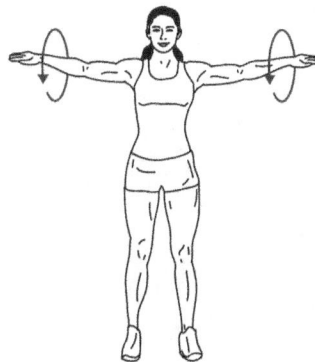

20 raised arm circles

20 march steps

Fitness is a journey, not a destination.
Darebee Project